Your Daily Happiness Boost

With 32 Sophrology Exercises and Other Tips 'n' Tricks

Jon Sofier & Judy Plume

Copyright © Jon Sofier & Judy Plume 2020

All rights reserved. This book is copyright material and must not be copied, reproduced, transferred, distributed, leased, licensed or used in any way except as specifically permitted in writing by the author, as allowed under the terms and conditions under which it was purchased or as strictly permitted by applicable copyright law. Respective authors own all copyrights not held by the publisher. In no way is it legal to reproduce, duplicate, or transmit any part of this document in either electronic means or printed format.

Any unauthorised distribution or use of this text may be a direct infringement of the Author's rights, and those responsible may be liable in law accordingly.

DISCLAIMER

The contents in this book are geared towards providing tested and reliable information about the topic and issue covered. While all attempts have been made to verify information provided in this publication, the Author and Publisher assume no responsibility for errors, omissions, or contrary interpretation of the subject matter herein.

The information herein is offered for educational, informational and reference purposes solely and is universal as so. It is not in any manner a substitute for professional medical advice or direct guidance of a qualified Sophrology instructor. Not all practices are suitable for all people. All readers are advised to seek services of competent professionals (Sophrology instructor or health care provider) before attempting to use any of the practices or information. Under no circumstances will any legal responsibility or blame be held against the Authors or publisher and they don't take any responsibility or liability for any injuries, reparation, damages or losses due to the information herein, either directly or indirectly.

The presentation of the information is without contract or any type of guarantee assurance. In practical advice books, like anything else in life, there are no guarantees of results. Readers are cautioned to rely on their judgment about their circumstances and act accordingly.

planetsophro.com

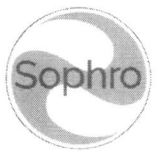

TABLE OF CONTENTS

DISCLAIMER	3
TABLE OF CONTENTS	5
INTRODUCTION	7
A FEW WORDS ON HAPPINESS	11
HOW SOPHROLOGY WORKS	13
A Proof for Sceptics – THE THUMB TRICK	15
Chapter 1: DITCH UNWANTED STRESS	17
The Fan	
Windmills	
Karate Kid	
Body Scan	
Breathe Out The Negative	
Chapter 2: GAIN PERSPECTIVE	31
Body Bubble	
Half And Half	
Trip Into Space	
Chapter 3: BE ZEN	41
Expanding Chest	
Welcome In	
Expanding Tummy	
Breathe In What You Need	
Chapter 4: BOOST YOUR FOCUS	51
The Third Eye	
Object Concentration	
Come To Your Senses	

Chapter 5: BOOST YOUR CONFIDENCE — 59
    The "No" Exercise
    The "Yes" Exercise
    Personal Gesture
    Pride From My Past

Chapter 6: BOOST YOUR ENERGY — 71
    Walk On The Spot
    Shoulder Pump
    Jumping Jack
    Waterfall Visualization
    Trip To The Sun

Chapter 7: SHINE AT ANY EVENT — 83
    Pre-Live Your Future Success

Chapter 8: FEEL THE NEW YOU — 89
    Feel Your Head
    Feel Your Arms
    Feel Your Legs
    Feel Your Body
    Sophro Mirror
    Back To The Future

THE THREE TECHNIQUES — 103
    Controlled Breathing
    Relaxed Movement Exercises
    Visualization

About The Founder: ALFONSO CAYCEDO — 105

SOURCES AND INSPIRATIONS — 107

INTRODUCTION

It's great to be happy, fulfilled and at peace. We hope that's what you're feeling right now! However we don't always feel good about ourselves.

How are you feeling right now? Take a moment to get in touch with yourself. Write down a few things you are feeling at the moment:

- _____
- _____
- _____

Are the adjectives you are feeling only positive? Or are there some negative ones too? If so, don't worry, you are not alone! In this book you will find solutions to help you alleviate the negative and accentuate the positive. The awareness you have of yourself is the basis for the journey we will be going on together.

Well-being is not a given. But it is within our power to achieve. It's possible to find things that make us feel good on a deeper, longer-lasting level, if we go looking for them and start appreciating them.

And with the help of our friend Woo, who you will meet soon, we will introduce you to Sophrology and give you some general tips, so we can all go together on the journey towards more happiness and well-being. If there are negative adjectives in your assessment above, we will tackle them with Woo!

One problem is that our brains naturally tend to the negative. This is a hard-wired trait from our distant past, designed to alert us against danger. Situations needed to be assessed quickly in order to keep us safe. It was better to assume a weirdly-shaped stick was a snake than to take a chance on getting harmed.

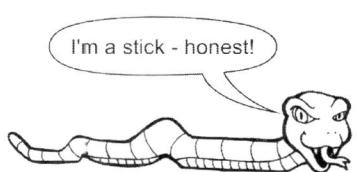

But we are no longer roaming the bushes and can do our bit to change this hard-wiring against these now not-so-present dangers.

The exercises in this book are drawn from Sophrology, a mind and body technique that mixes Western science and Eastern practices. We hope you become best friends with these exercises as you learn to feel better and better about yourself. Even if you take a break from them for a while, they will still be there for you. And it will feel like you have never been apart.

Why your best friend?

Because the exercises:

- Are always there for you.
- Make you feel good and give you a boost.
- Accompany you, support you and help you understand yourself.

In order to feel more positive, we don't need to avoid all the negative things in our lives. That would be impossible anyway. We need to encourage the positive things which will, little by little, take the place of the negative. Psychologist Ed Diener suggested that well-being does not come from one massive positive experience that changes the way we see the world. It comes from lots of little positive events in our lives. The frequency is more important than the intensity.

The Sophrology exercises in this book are part of these little positive events!

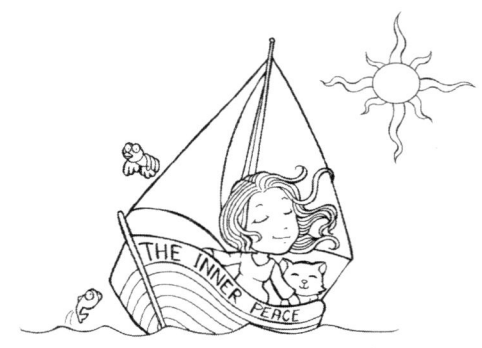

Sometimes we can feel a bit like ships, riding the waves. We all sail through rough conditions from time to time. We find sleep difficult and toss 'n' turn in bed, as if we were being battered by the sea and the weather. Daily chores and events affect our state of mind, even when we are at rest. It's necessary at times to change tack completely and head for calmer waters. Like Woo and her friends, we can find a bay, shelter from the storm and relax in the sun to recharge our batteries. Even if it's just for a few minutes a day. Sophrology is like this bay. It's a place to go in order to replenish our forces. Or just relax for a bit.

Furthermore it's not selfish to recognise that we are the most important person in our lives. So it's crucial to look after ourselves. It's virtually impossible to change the world massively, but we can change ourselves and learn how to deal better with situations. And if we change, sometimes others change too. If we're happy inside, we're likely to spread happiness. If we feel bad we're likely to spread negativity.

So remember, when it comes to well-being, it's not just for your own good, but also for the good of others and the world!

Psychologist and Nobel Prize winner Daniel Kahneman observed that, "When it comes to well-being attention is key, that our emotional state is largely determined by what we attend to and what we are focused on." So we need to focus on ourselves from time to time!

Treat this book like your best friend! Put it somewhere where you have access to it at all times! Then use it whenever you are in need.

What the chapters offer:

We kick off by giving a few thoughts on happiness and then we move onto a short introduction of Sophrology. Before the exercise chapters, we show you a cool trick on how powerful our minds can be.

- The first three chapters look at different ways to deal with unwanted stress. Distress, as the experts call it, which we often put on ourselves. So we are looking at how to ditch unwanted stress, gain perspective and how to train ourselves to be zen.
- Next we want to bring in more positivity. In the following three chapters we reinforce our capabilities. We are looking to improve concentration, boost our energy levels and build up confidence.
- After that, we get real and help you prepare mentally for an event, which could be a job interview, sports event or even preparing for giving birth. The challenges for important events in our lives are similar and we'd like you to shine at all of them!
- Finally we want you to take a look and be proud of how far you have come. The objective of the last chapter "Feel the New You" is to make you realise all the positive changes you have made.
- Note: Throughout the chapters there are intention boxes to help you consider your daily challenges and aspirations as you do the exercises.

At the end of the book you learn about the basic tools of Sophrology. You will also find out about Alfonso Caycedo and how/why he created Sophrology.

You can start with the exercises in the order presented in this book. They are arranged for a person who is new to Sophrology. Alternatively you can delve into this book at random or concentrate on your favourite chapters. The chapters are interchangeable and interdependent. Why? Because everything is connected.

For example we need to be calm to concentrate and concentrate to be calm. Try to get to know the exercises and the effects they have. Repeat as often as you can, because that's how you'll integrate them. Some exercises can be done seated and almost invisibly if you are in an office or on public transport. For others you will need a bit of time and space for yourself. The time and space you deserve! Like your new best friend, these exercises will become a part of you.

Here are some final tips before you get started:

- Imagine leaving your problems on a coat hanger by the door as you do the exercises. The problems will still be there, but for now you can forget them as you spend some much-deserved time on you.
- Imagine the time spent on the exercises as a little parentheses in your day.
- Accept all the feelings you have during the exercises with loving-kindness and without judgment, just like a best friend would.
- It's normal for your mind to wander. If it does, gently bring it back to the exercise you're doing.
- Never criticise yourself. In fact...
- Thank and congratulate yourself for spending this time and effort on you!

We wish you a lot of fun with this book and the exercises. We hope you will enjoy getting to know a new best friend!

A FEW WORDS ON HAPPINESS

The universe was not created simply to make us happy, unfortunately!

The idea that happiness should be a constant state of mind is of course wishful thinking. If we were happy all the time we would never learn, never tap into our resourcefulness or develop creativity. This would be detrimental to our species. We would merely be robots and wouldn't that be sad!

But of course we all want to be as happy as possible for the short period of time we spend on this planet. So how can we achieve that? We can learn to value, treasure and celebrate all the emotions we experience, even the bad ones. They are a gift. They help us distinguish. They help us question. They help us progress into creating who we really want to be. We gradually learn to do more of the things that make us happy and less of the things that make us unhappy.

We are all the same in the sense that we are all made out of the same stuff and hardwiring. Most of us have similar goals like pursuing partnerships, success and happiness. Yet we are different because we don't all feel and think about these things in the same way. In order to create our personal happiness boosters we need to find out how we feel and think about all of those things.

Happiness is complex and elusive. It's made out of bits and pieces. And those bits and pieces need attention because they change over time. It is a constant work in progress if you like.

That's where self-awareness comes into play. Training in observing how we think, feel and behave. Trying to glean as much information about ourselves as possible. With that information we can then create our little bits of happiness to implement in our daily lives.

Sophrology is very useful here. The aim of Sophrology is to increase our self-awareness and give ourselves what we need in order to advance and become more fulfilled.

There's no one single definition of happiness. But it's always good to collect as many relaxed and happy moments as possible.

It's equally important to recognise that unless there is a mental illness at play, happiness is a choice, not something that just happens. Choose Sophrology to add to the number of positive experiences in your life!

Super effective and unashamedly positive!

HOW SOPHROLOGY WORKS

If, like us, you're a fan of yoga, meditation, NLP and talk therapy, Sophrology might be the thing for you. It is complementary to all of them and it is also a discipline in its own right.

- It's a method that combines body and mind in order to help us develop. It has the advantages of a yoga session but we don't have to change our clothes or do anything too physical. It has the advantages of meditation and we are guided by a Sophrologist throughout the session, or this little book! It includes visualizations that we find in NLP, which help us take resources from our past, enjoy our present and be excited about our future. And it can combine with talk-based therapies to help us live our new answers physically, not just mentally.

- It's like a best friend that supports us in all areas of our lives. Sophrology focuses on the positive. It digs into our tastes and preferences, the resources and capacities in our lives that bring us joy. The general idea is to use Relaxed Movement exercises and visualizations to become more aware mentally and physically – which in return helps us solve problems, bring positivity and happiness.

- It builds up resources to call upon whenever we need them. If we are in a difficult situation it might seem bizarre at first to reconnect with positivity and joy. Because this needs to be learned. Try to remember when you started riding a bike. Did the little you secretly doubt at the beginning that balancing on that thing would really work? But after a while it did and now it's hard to imagine that it ever seemed difficult. With Sophrology, we learn to anchor our positive outcome through repetition. Once that is achieved we find it easier to put ourselves into that state of mind again when we need it.

The things that are important here are how we feel, what we feel and how we perceive our world, without internal judgments about these feelings. With Sophrology we are given the tools to observe and develop our emotions and feel the impact on our bodies - or vice versa - in other words to observe and develop our bodies and feel the impact on our emotions.

A Proof for Sceptics – THE THUMB TRICK

If you are sceptical about the power of the mind on the body, try this little fun exercise!

Stand upright, with your arm outstretched in front of your face and your thumb pointing upwards as if you were hitch-hiking. Focus your eyes on your thumb. Now rotate your body as far as it will go in one direction. You will certainly be able to turn more than 180°. Once you have gone as far as you can, fix a point in the background in line with your thumb so you remember how much your body rotated. Return to your starting position.

Now close your eyes and in your mind imagine rotating your body as far as possible. Then go even further! Think about going through a full 360°! And then keep going! Imagine rotating your body through another 360° to make 720°!

Open your eyes and try the exercise once more in reality. Rotate your body as far as it will go. Fix a point in the background again and compare it to your previous attempt. How much further did you get this time?

Sportspeople use this exercise to help them surpass their previous best performances.

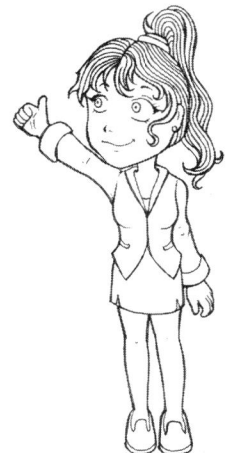
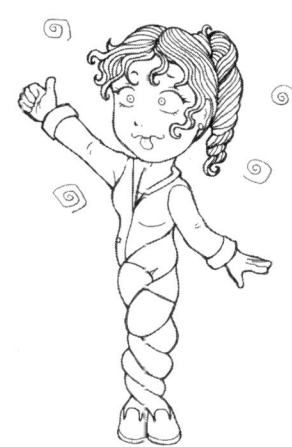

Chapter 1: DITCH UNWANTED STRESS

Some stress (known as good stress or eustress) is linked to healthy challenges and helps us advance. On the other hand bad stress or distress aggravates illnesses, psychological diseases and disturbs our relationships. We're calling this Unwanted Stress.

This kind of stress has an addictive nature. It's caused by stressful events that in return cause anxiety which again causes stress. Until it turns chronic when our bodies get constantly flooded with stress hormones, like cortisol. If we want to stay healthy we need to avoid that. Everybody has to deal with these events in their lives. It could be the loss of a job, a break-up or a traumatic event like the death of a loved one. These are external stress factors and we all have to go through them.

But here's the thing, a lot of people suffer from internal stress, like worries. Worries can grow bigger and turn into full-blown anxiety and illness.

Whatever you worry about, we love this study by Robert Leahy, which showed that 85% of our worries never actually happen. And of the 15% that do happen, 79% of the subjects decided afterwards that they handled the situation better than they expected. So about 97% of what we worry and stress about is completely useless!

So let's shake it off and get rid of it.

Maybe you have experienced that it is not useful to tell yourself to stop stressing. It's like saying, "Try not to think of an elephant!" And what do you think about?

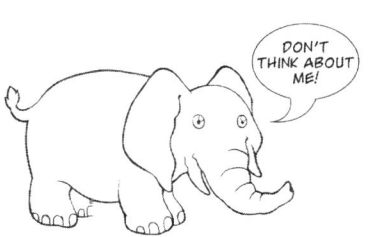

So that doesn't work. But the following does:

- It's better to take the mind and body to a completely different place.
- Get away. Change scenery. Preferably outside, where you can enjoy nature. And if that's not possible, do a nature visualization.

- Trigger your body's positive response by smiling until you feel it, even if you don't feel it at the beginning. Your brain will send out the corresponding emotional response. Or you can simply watch a comedy you like.

- Chew something, preferably a chewing gum. The chewing movement and taste have a calming effect on us.

- Do some kind of active sport. Not new information but still a good stress reliever and worth mentioning.

- Many people advocate meditation, good breathing and exercise for countering unwanted stress. Sophrology combines elements of all three of these things in its exercises. It is particularly well-adapted to getting rid of unwanted stress. Use Relaxed Movement exercises like "The Fan", "Karate Kid" and "Windmills". The two visualization exercises are the "Body Scan", to bring yourself back home to you, and "Breathe Out The Negative" to release the tensions from your body.

Setting Intentions

Reflect on and write down situations currently giving you stress:

- _____
- _____
- _____

As you do the exercises keep these stresses in mind. Set the intention of eliminating them as you do the exercises!

The Fan

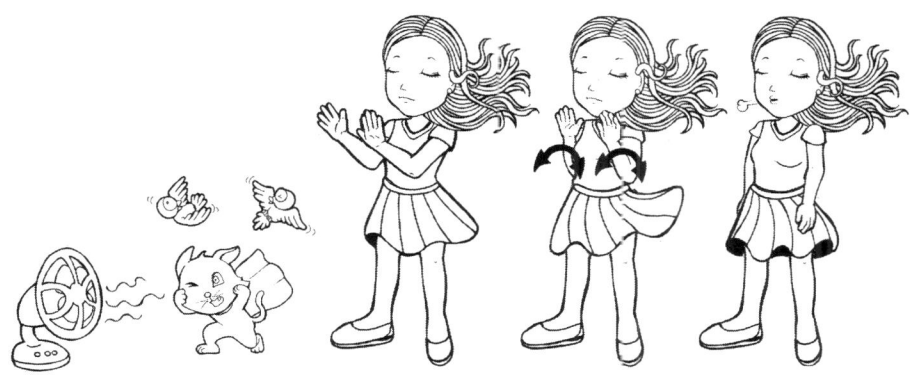

Stand up

Close your eyes.

Lift up your arms to the horizontal level.

Breathe in through your nose and hold your breath.

Shake your hands like two fans as you bring them back towards your chest.

Imagine wiping away your stress.

Breathe out through your mouth as you let your arms fall by your side.

Breathe naturally again.

Notice your sensations.

Think about your arms, your hands.

Become aware of the relaxed feelings in your arms and hands.

Do the exercise a second time.

Lift up your arms to the horizontal level.

Breathe in through your nose and hold your breath.

Shake your hands like two fans as you bring them back towards your chest.

Imagine shaking away your stress.

Breathe out through your mouth as you let your arms fall by your side.

Breathe naturally again.

Notice your sensations.

Think about the movement of your arms and hands.

Become aware that you have shaken away your stress.

Do the exercise a third time.

Lift up your arms to the horizontal level.

Breathe in through your nose and hold your breath.

Shake your hands like two fans as you bring them back towards your chest.

Imagine getting rid of all your stress.

Breathe out through your mouth as you let your arms fall by your side.

Breathe naturally again.

Notice your sensations.

Welcome all your feelings.

Become aware of your capacity to shake off your stress.

The exercise is now finished and you can open your eyes.

Windmills

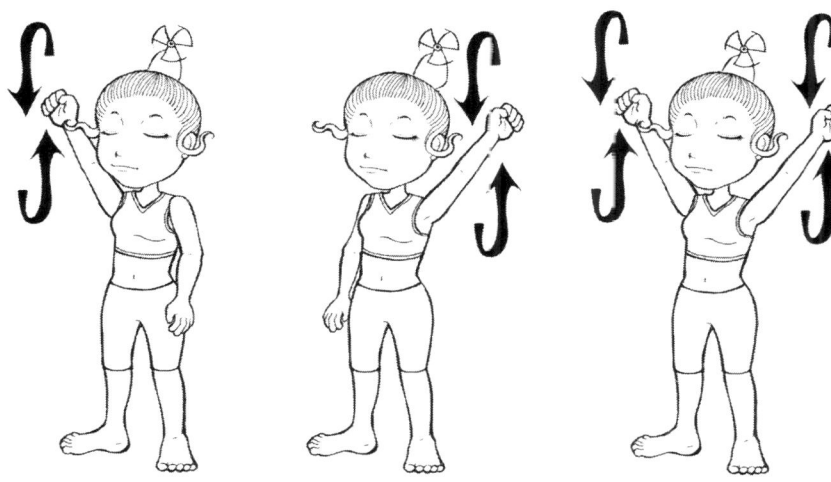

Stand up.

Close your eyes.

Breathe in through your nose and hold your breath.

Rotate your right arm round and round several times.

Picture a problem and imagine throwing it away.

Let your arm come back by your side as you breathe out through your mouth.

Breathe naturally again.

Notice your sensations.

Welcome the feelings in your right arm.

Become aware of the relaxation in your right arm.

Do the same exercise with your left arm.

Breathe in through your nose and hold your breath.

Rotate your left arm round and round several times.

Imagine throwing away your tensions.

Let your arm come back by your side as you breathe out through your mouth.

Breathe naturally again.

Notice your sensations.

Feel the relaxation in your left arm.

Become aware that you have thrown away your tensions.

Do the exercise a third time with both arms.

Breathe in through your nose and hold your breath.

Rotate both your arms round and round several times.

Imagine throwing away all your stress.

Let your arms come back by your side as you breathe out through your mouth.

Breathe naturally again.

Notice your sensations.

Welcome all your feelings.

Become aware of your capacity to throw away your stress.

The exercise is now finished and you can open your eyes.

Karate Kid

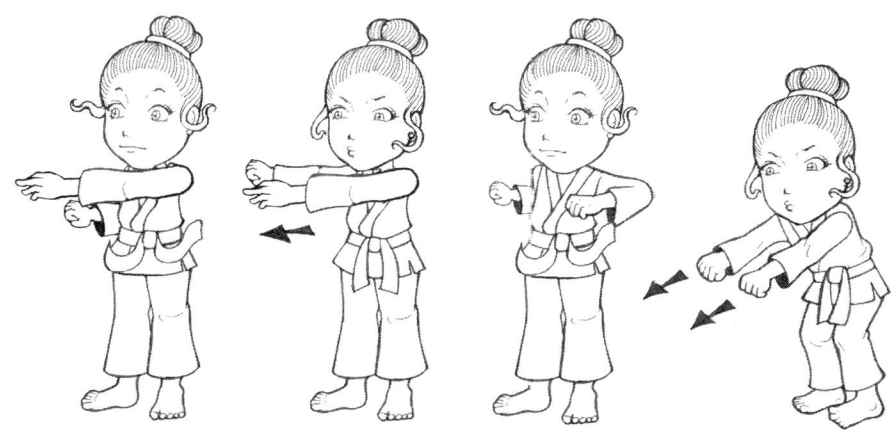

Stand up.

Keep your eyes open.

Lift up your left arm to the horizontal position.

Bring your right fist to the height of your right shoulder with your elbow pointing backwards.

Breathe in through your nose and hold your breath.

Pick an imaginary point opposite you as a target and imagine it contains your problems.

Launch your right fist towards it, exhaling loudly through your mouth.

Breathe naturally again as you relax your arms by your side.

Close your eyes and notice your sensations.

Feel the sensations in your arms.

Become aware of the power of your gesture.

Open your eyes and do the exercise a second time, with the other arm.

Lift up your right arm to the horizontal position.

Bring your left fist to the height of your left shoulder with your elbow pointing backwards.

Breathe in through your nose and hold your breath.

Pick an imaginary point opposite you as a target and imagine it contains your stress.

Launch your left fist towards it, exhaling loudly through your mouth.

Breathe naturally again as you relax your arms by your side.

Close your eyes and notice your sensations.

Feel the precision of your gesture.

Become aware that you have destroyed your stress.

Open your eyes and do the exercise a third time with both arms.

Bring both fists to the height of your shoulders with your elbows pointing backwards.

Breathe in through your nose and hold your breath.

Pick an imaginary point opposite you as a target and imagine it contains your tensions.

Launch your fists towards it, exhaling loudly through your mouth.

Breathe naturally again as you relax your arms by your side.

Close your eyes and notice your sensations.

Welcome all your feelings.

Become aware of your capacity to destroy your tensions.

The exercise is now finished and you can open your eyes.

Body Scan

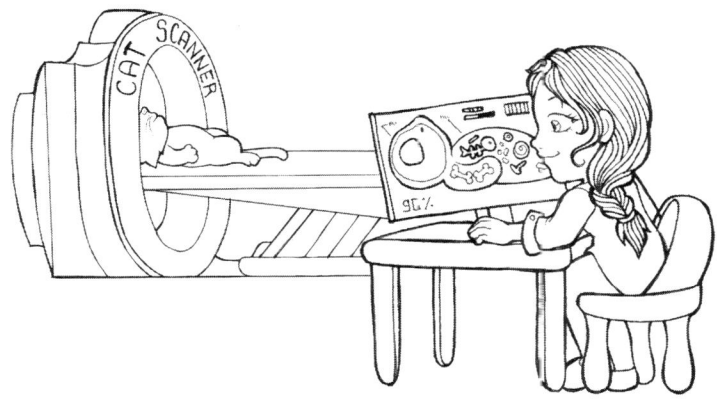

Sit down.

Close your eyes.

Start by feeling all the contact points on your body.

Feel your back and bottom against the chair.

Your hands on your thighs.

Your feet on the ground.

Feel the air against your face.

Become aware of the calmness that is flowing through your body.

Bring your attention to your head and face.

Think about the top of your head, your forehead and temples.

Relax your eyes in their sockets.

Relax your cheeks and nose.

Feel the fresh air entering your nostrils with each in-breath.

Feel the warmer air exiting your nostrils as you breathe out.

Relax your mouth and jaws.

Let your tongue lie naturally in your mouth.

Think about your ears.

Become aware that your head and face are now relaxed.

Allow this relaxation to spread into your neck and shoulders.

Let it diffuse into your arms.

Feel the relaxation spread down your arms, through your elbows and forearms.

Relax your wrists, hands and fingers - right to the end of your fingertips.

Become aware that your shoulders, arms and hands are now completely relaxed.

Turn your attention to your back.

Relax your back from the top to the bottom.

Feel your spine and relax all the muscles connected to it.

Become aware that your back is now completely relaxed.

Bring your attention to your chest.

Feel it move as you breathe in and out.

Observe your rib cage rising with each inhale and falling with each exhale.

Notice the beating of your heart.

Feel the movements of your abdomen, rising and falling a bit like waves on a beach.

Feel your stomach relax.

Relax your hips, your bottom, your sexual organs.

Become aware that your torso is now completely relaxed.

Let this relaxation spread into your legs.

Relax all the muscles in your legs from the thighs, through the knees, to the calves, ankles and feet.

Feel the relaxation pass to the tips of your toenails.

Become aware that your legs and feet are now completely relaxed.

Become aware that your whole body is now completely relaxed.

Remember that these relaxed feelings are always present in you.

Think about activating them in your daily life when you feel stressed.

The exercise is now finished and you can open your eyes.

Breathe Out The Negative

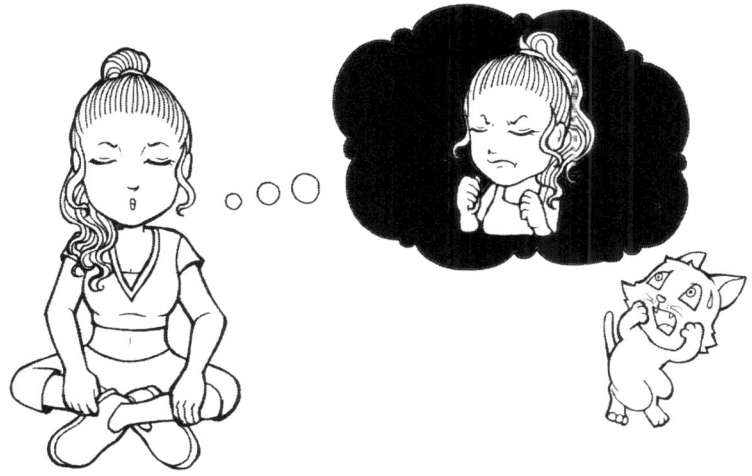

Sit down.

Close your eyes.

Feel all the contact points on your body.

Feel your back and bottom against the chair.

Your hands on your thighs.

Your feet on the ground.

Feel the air against your face.

Become aware of the calmness that is flowing through your body.

Take a deep breath and tense up all the muscles in your body.

Hold your breath and keep all your muscles contracted.

Now exhale strongly and relax these muscles, releasing the stresses and tensions from your body.

Breathe naturally again.

Become aware of the relaxation spreading through your body.

Bring your attention to your head and face.

Notice the areas where you feel tense.

Breathe in and contract the muscles in your head and face that feel tense.

Hold your breath and keep these muscles contracted.

Now exhale strongly and relax all these muscles, releasing the stresses and tensions from your head and face.

Breathe naturally again.

Become aware of the relaxation spreading through your head and face.

Bring your attention to your neck, shoulders and arms.

Notice the areas where you feel tense.

Breathe in and contract the muscles in your neck, shoulders and arms that feel tense.

Hold your breath and keep these muscles contracted.

Now exhale strongly and relax all these muscles, releasing the stresses and tensions from your neck, shoulders and arms.

Breathe naturally again.

Become aware of the relaxation spreading through your neck, shoulders and arms.

Bring your attention to your back.

Notice the areas where you feel tense.

Breathe in and contract the muscles in your back that feel tense.

Hold your breath and keep these muscles contracted.

Now exhale strongly and relax all these muscles, releasing the stresses and tensions from your back.

Breathe naturally again.

Become aware of the relaxation spreading through your back.

Bring your attention to the rest of your torso.

Notice the areas where you feel tense.

Breathe in and contract the muscles of your torso that feel tense.

Hold your breath and keep these muscles contracted.

Now exhale strongly and relax all these muscles, releasing the stresses and tensions from your torso.

Breathe naturally again.

Become aware of the relaxation spreading through your torso.

Bring your attention to your legs and feet.

Notice the areas where you feel tense.

Breathe in and contract the muscles in your legs and feet that feel tense.

Hold your breath and keep these muscles contracted.

Now exhale strongly and relax all these muscles, releasing the stresses and tensions from your legs and feet.

Breathe naturally again.

Become aware of the relaxation spreading through your legs and feet.

Finally take a deep breath and tense up all the muscles in your body once more.

Hold your breath and keep all these muscles contracted.

Now exhale strongly and relax these muscles, releasing all the remaining stresses and tensions from your body.

Breathe naturally again.

Become aware of the relaxation spreading through your body.

Remember that these feelings are always present in you.

Think about them in your daily life when you want to relax.

The exercise is now finished and you can open your eyes.

Chapter 2: GAIN PERSPECTIVE

Ok, so you think you're in a shitty situation that you can't get out of, money problems, job troubles, conflicts with your partner. Maybe you feel inundated by the news or things that aren't going your way. However hard you try it seems you cannot escape your problems.

You are like the fly that is trapped inside a room, desperately trying to find its way out. It goes backwards and forwards, only to bump into the same spot again and again. Sometimes this goes on for hours as it makes the irritating buzzing noise that we all know so well. Until, finally, the fly tries a different angle and finds its way out.

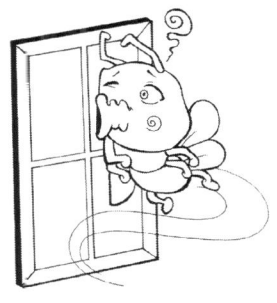

Sometimes we are like that fly. We try to tackle a problem with an approach that has already failed time and again.

Whether you are facing a one-time problem or it's something that you feel you are repeatedly confronted with, here are some tips on how to overcome them and gain some perspective:

- Look at your belief systems. Is there an IF ... , THEN ... belief that causes you problems? Belief systems are difficult to approach since they have often been ingrained in us from when we were little. We learn from childhood that they are true and feel comfortable with them, until, well, now. This can be quite tricky, since we don't always see ourselves clearly, so you might need the help of a therapist.

If you find some belief systems on your own, check they are actually true for you. If not change them! That sounds easy but it's really hard. A belief system has to be unlearned and replaced by practising and learning to feel comfortable with the new one. The one that is true for you now! Here are two common examples of belief systems that we are talking about: «If I am not available all the time, then I am not a good friend» or «If I don't look like the woman in the magazine, then I won't find love.» There are plenty more! Belief systems are as unique as people!

- Take time out of the equation. When you think about the fly that is bumping into the window over and over again, don't you wish it would just fly further away so that it could see the gap in the window? Give yourself some time and space to find the gap for your specific problem!

"Distance lends enchantment to the view," wrote Mark Twain. Or to put it another more colourful way, if our head is stuck inside a big pile of shit, we may not be able to find many useful answers. Things do not look good from that perspective!

If we're too close to our problems, we can't see the wood for the trees. The ideal thing might be to take a long holiday on a paradisiacal island in order to put things into perspective. But maybe we don't have the time or the money for such a solution. Luckily Sophrology is here to help.

- The exercises in this chapter are designed to help us see things from a distance. With the Relaxed Movement exercise, "Body Bubble", we're encouraged to create a little bubble around us so we're less affected by what happens close to us. The exercise "Half and Half" encourages us to see our situation with perspective. We are looking down on our problems from above.

Going on a Sophrological "Trip into Space" is in itself a magical experience. And on your "return" to Earth you may have a different perspective on things.

Taking a step back from any situation is usually beneficial. It teaches us that our problems don't define us. We can detach ourselves from our troubles and treat them as passing events.

Let Sophrology help you do this! It is there to help you, whether your problem is real or imagined, big or small!

Setting Intentions

Reflect on and write down any problems and emotions you would like to put into perspective:

- _____
- _____
- _____

As you do the exercises keep these problems and emotions in mind. Set the intention of seeing them differently as you do the exercises!

Body Bubble

Setting Intention

As you do this exercise, set the intention of creating a protective bubble around you.

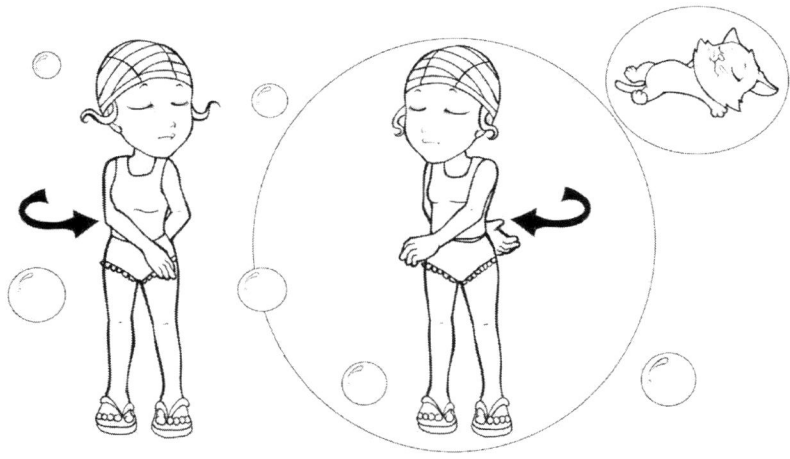

Stand up.

Close your eyes.

Breathe in through your nose and hold your breath.

Rotate your body around your spine, letting your arms and head follow the movement.

Imagine the area all around you.

Breathe out through your mouth while returning to your starting position.

Breathe naturally again.

Notice your sensations.

Welcome the feelings in your arms and head.

Become aware of the space all around you.

Do the exercise a second time.

Breathe in through your nose and hold your breath.

Rotate your body around your spine, letting your arms and head follow the movement.

Imagine you're creating a space all around you.

Breathe out through your mouth while returning to your starting position.

Breathe naturally again.

Notice your sensations.

Welcome the feelings of relaxation in your arms and head.

Become aware of creating a space around you.

Do the exercise a third time.

Breathe in through your nose and hold your breath.

Rotate your body around your spine, letting your arms and head follow the movement.

Imagine you've created a protective bubble all around you.

Breathe out through your mouth while returning to your starting position.

Breathe naturally again.

Notice your sensations.

Welcome all your feelings.

Become aware of your capacity to create a protective bubble around you.

The exercise is now finished and you can open your eyes.

Half And Half

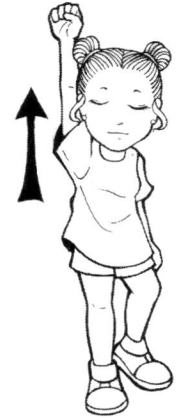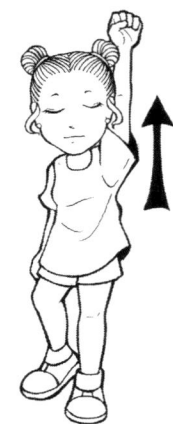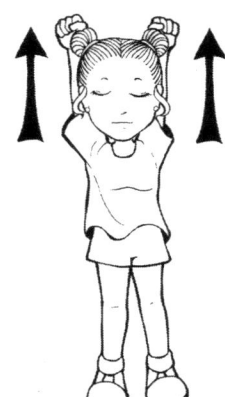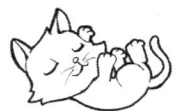

Stand up.

Close your eyes.

Move your weight onto your right foot.

Raise your right arm in the air.

Breathe in through your nose and hold your breath.

Stretch the right-hand side of your body by raising your right hand towards the sky.

Imagine pushing your problems away from you.

Breathe out through your mouth while letting your right arm fall by your side.

Return to a normal standing position and breathe naturally again.

Notice your sensations.

Feel the sensations in the right half of your body.

Become aware of the worries that you have pushed away from you.

Do the exercise a second time with your left arm.

Move your weight onto your left foot.

Raise your left arm into the air.

Breathe in through your nose and hold your breath.

Stretch the left-hand side of your body by raising your left hand towards the sky.

Imagine seeing yourself from a higher perspective.

Breathe out through your mouth while letting your left arm fall by your side.

Return to a normal standing position and breathe naturally again.

Notice your sensations.

Feel the sensations in the left half of your body.

Become aware of seeing things from a new height.

Do the exercise a third time with both arms.

Raise both arms into the air.

Breathe in through your nose and hold your breath.

Stretch your body by raising your hands towards the sky.

Imagine seeing yourself from a new angle.

Breathe out through your mouth while letting your arms fall by your side.

Breathe naturally again.

Notice your sensations.

Welcome all your feelings.

Become aware of your capacity to see yourself from a new angle.

The exercise is now finished and you can open your eyes.

Trip Into Space

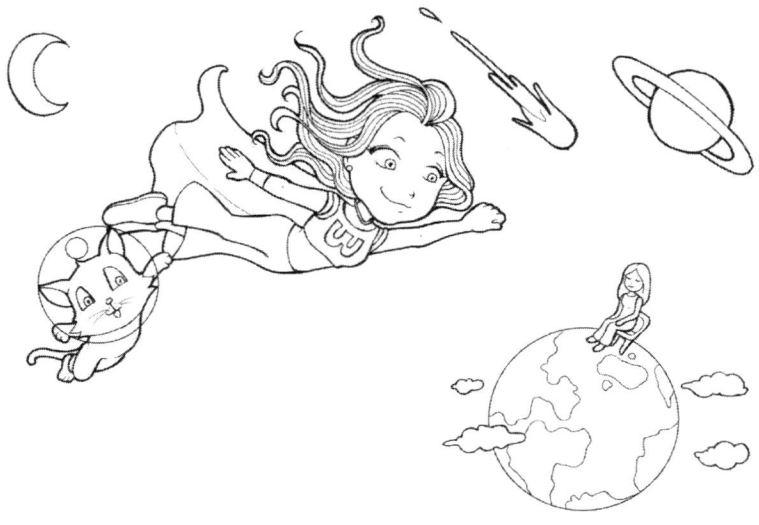

Sit down.

Close your eyes and imagine your body.

Picture yourself where you are right now.

Now look down on yourself from above.

Visualize your body as you continue your ascension.

See the place where you live.

Imagine your town and region.

Picture your country with its borders.

Think now about the continents and the seas.

Continue your ascension.

You can now see the whole of the Earth.

Visualize all the colours and shapes of our planet.

Contemplate its beauty.

Now go on a trip to see the rest of the planets in the solar system.

Turn your attention to the stars and galaxies.

Admire all the beauties of our immense Universe.

Fully live this incredible moment.

Prepare yourself to slowly come back down to Earth.

Take in once more the beauty of our planet from space.

Begin your descent.

See the continents and the oceans

Take your time to admire their beauty.

Picture your country with its borders and features.

Slowly continue your descent.

Visualize your region and the area where you live.

Pick out the place where you currently are.

Look down on your body from above.

Observe its calmness and serenity.

Fully integrate these sensations.

Remember that these feelings are always present in you.

Think about them in your daily life when you need to see things with more perspective.

The exercise is now finished and you can open your eyes.

Chapter 3: BE ZEN

What would you describe as a crisis situation? Under what circumstances do you go into an emotional upheaval? And more importantly what do you do then?

Even though you probably have a different definition and reaction to crisis from us, everybody sometimes reacts out of distress and panic. We go into our ancient hardwired behaviour of fight, flight or freeze. Without thinking we react in a counterproductive manner. Maybe you agree that getting it right or totally mucking up a situation sometimes just depends on your state of mind.

That's where calm comes into play, in order to help us unmuck something. Ok, we agree it's not always easy to get out of confusion and agitation, but it is trainable and learnable. And it's worth it. It helps us make better choices, reduce suffering and maintain good health, mentally and physically.

- Generally you can unwind by simply counting to 10. When you are amongst people this will also add a certain dramatic effect, as they have to curiously wait for your response.

- Taking a few deep breaths when in panic mode can chase away the demons. If you have the chance you can combine that with doing a few Sophrology exercises.

- So let's get started with a bit of Sophrology to find that special calm place, that you can always revisit when there is chaos all around you. You inhale this calmness with the exercise, "Breathe in What You Need." And with the Relaxed Movement exercises you welcome it in and spread it through and around your body.

Note: The first three chapters in this book on stress, perspective and calm are so dependent on each other that it's sometimes hard to separate them. What's essential here is to see that you generally want to get rid of any stress and bring in the calm and perspective. It's amazing how much more positive energy we have when the crap is gone!

> **Setting Intention**
>
> As you do the exercises set the intention of increasing your overall calmness!

Expanding Chest

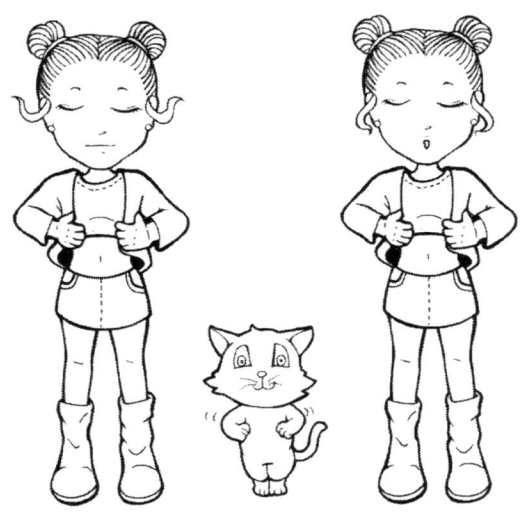

Stand up.

Close your eyes.

Put your hands on your ribs.

Expand your chest by breathing in deeply through your nose.

Imagine calmness entering your body.

Breathe out gently through your mouth and feel your chest decrease in size.

Breathe naturally again.

Notice your sensations.

Feel your chest opening and broadening.

Become aware of the movement of your chest.

Do the exercise a second time.

Expand your chest by breathing in deeply through your nose.

Imagine spreading calmness throughout your body.

Breathe out gently through your mouth and feel your chest decrease in size.

Breathe naturally again.

Notice your sensations.

Feel the suppleness of your chest

Become aware of the calmness that you've breathed into your body.

Do the exercise a third time.

Expand your chest by breathing in deeply through your nose.

Imagine taking calmness into your body.

Breathe out gently through your mouth and feel your chest decrease in size.

Breathe naturally again.

Let your arms fall by your side and notice your sensations.

Welcome all your feelings.

Become aware of your capacity to breathe calmness into your body.

The exercise is now finished and you can open your eyes.

Welcome In

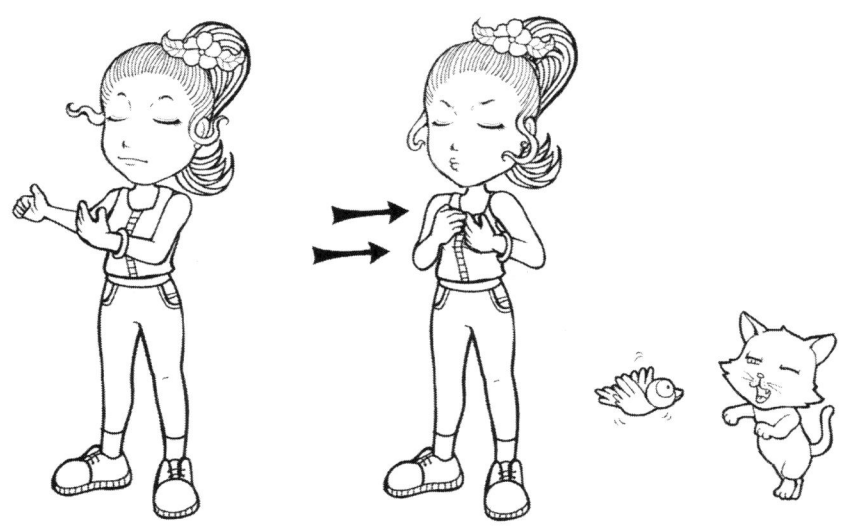

Stand up.

Close your eyes.

Lift your arms to the horizontal position with your hands open.

Breathe in through your nose and hold your breath.

Slowly bring your hands towards your chest.

Imagine calmness entering your body.

Breathe out through your mouth as you relax your arms by your side.

Breathe naturally again.

Notice your sensations.

Feel the sensations in your arms and hands.

Become aware of the movement of your arms.

Do the exercise a second time.

Lift your arms to the horizontal position with your hands open.

Breathe in through your nose and hold your breath.

Slowly bring your hands towards your chest.

Imagine bringing calmness into your body.

Breathe out through your mouth as you relax your arms by your side.

Breathe naturally again.

Notice your sensations.

Feel the relaxation in your arms.

Become aware of the calmness that you've welcomed into your body.

Do the exercise a third time.

Lift your arms to the horizontal position with your hands open.

Breathe in through your nose and hold your breath.

Slowly bring your hands towards your chest.

Imagine welcoming calmness into your body.

Breathe out through your mouth as you relax your arms by your side.

Breathe naturally again.

Notice your sensations.

Welcome all your feelings.

Become aware of your capacity to welcome calmness into your body.

The exercise is now finished and you can open your eyes.

Expanding Tummy

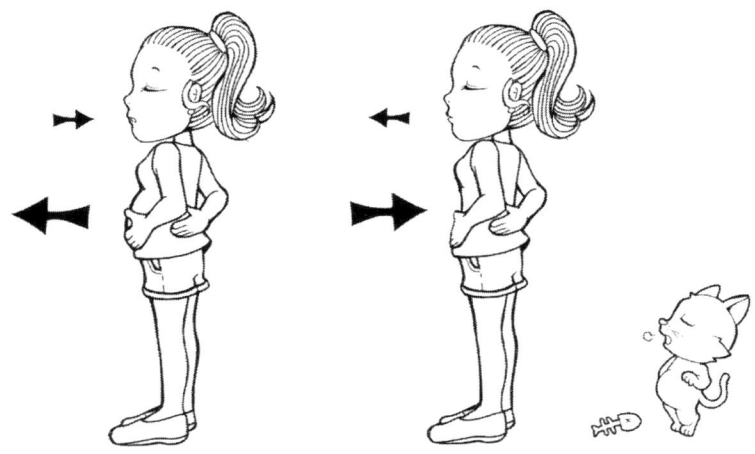

Stand up.

Close your eyes.

Put one hand on your tummy and the other on the small of your back.

Expand your tummy by breathing in deeply through your nose.

Imagine calmness entering your body.

Breathe out gently through your mouth and feel your tummy decreasing in size.

Breathe naturally again.

Notice your sensations.

Feel the suppleness of your stomach.

Become aware of the movement of your stomach.

Do the exercise a second time.

Expand your tummy by breathing in deeply through your nose.

Imagine spreading calmness throughout your body.

Breathe out gently through your mouth and feel your tummy decreasing in size.

Breathe naturally again.

Notice your sensations.

Feel your tummy area relax.

Become aware of the calmness spreading through your body.

Do the exercise a third time.

Expand your tummy by breathing in deeply through your nose.

Imagine diffusing calmness throughout your body.

Breathe out gently through your mouth and feel your tummy decreasing in size.

Breathe naturally again.

Let your arms fall by your side and notice your sensations.

Welcome all your feelings.

Become aware of your capacity to diffuse calmness throughout your body.

The exercise is now finished and you can open your eyes.

Breathe In What You Need

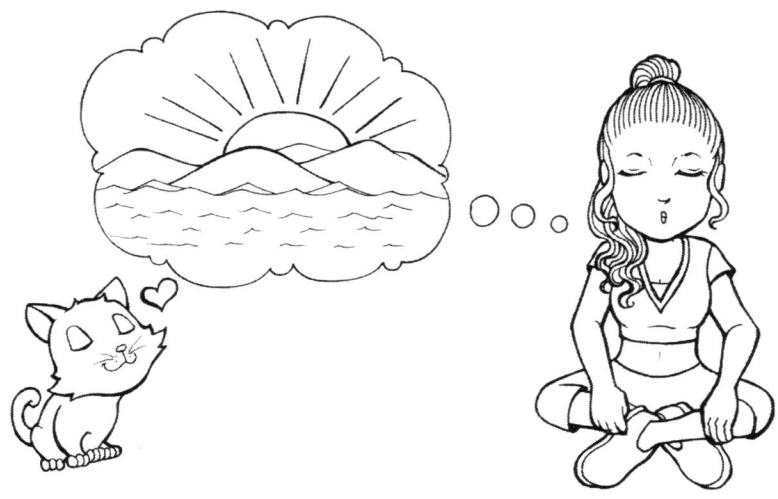

Sit down and close your eyes.

I want you to bring to your mind a happy, peaceful moment that you've lived.

Really feel that moment.

Live it as if it were now.

Let it inhabit your body.

Feel the sensations.

Now inhale deeply and take in even more of this positive moment.

Hold your breath.

And as you slowly breathe out, diffuse these feelings throughout your body.

Let the calmness spread from your head to your toes.

Breathe naturally again.

Notice the peaceful sensations throughout your body.

You're now going to do the same thing for all the different parts of your body.

Start with your head and face.

Inhale deeply and take in even more of this calm, peaceful moment.

Hold your breath.

As you slowly breathe out, diffuse these feelings throughout your head and face like a wave.

Let the sensations spread from the top of your head, through all of your face.

Breathe naturally again.

Notice all the peace and calmness in your head and face.

Now bring your attention to your shoulders, arms and hands.

Inhale deeply and take in some more of this calm, peaceful moment.

Hold your breath.

As you slowly breathe out, diffuse these feelings throughout your shoulders, arms and hands.

Let the sensations spread from your shoulders down through your arms and hands to the tips of your fingernails.

Breathe naturally again.

Notice all the peace and calmness in your shoulders, arms and hands.

Bring your attention to your torso.

Inhale deeply and take in more of this calm, peaceful moment.

Hold your breath.

As you slowly breathe out, diffuse these feelings throughout your back, chest and stomach.

Let the sensations spread from the top of your back, down your spine to your lower back region.

Feel the relaxation in your chest and stomach.

Breathe naturally again.

Notice all the peace and calmness in your back, chest and stomach.

Bring your attention to your hips, legs and feet.

Inhale deeply and take in this calm, peaceful moment once more.

Hold your breath.

As you slowly breathe out, diffuse these feelings throughout your hips, legs and feet.

Let the sensations spread from your hips and thighs, through your knees and calves, down through your ankles and feet to the tips of your toenails.

Breathe naturally again.

Notice all the peace and calmness in these parts of your body.

Finally inhale deeply one last time and take in even more of this positive moment.

Hold your breath.

As you slowly breathe out, diffuse these feelings throughout your whole body.

Let the calmness spread from your head to your toes.

Breathe naturally again.

Notice the peaceful sensations throughout your body.

Remember that these feelings are always present in you.

Think about them in your daily life when you want to feel calm and at peace.

The exercise is now finished and you can open your eyes.

Chapter 4: BOOST YOUR FOCUS

Do you have a mind that sometimes goes off at tangents? Do you worry about things at random? If so, you're far from alone. It's something our species seems to have done since the dawn of time. The Buddha spoke about the "Monkey Mind", a concept that probably existed before him. The idea is that our minds are like drunken monkeys, chattering and screeching while jumping around randomly. We need to calm those damn monkeys because the ability to concentrate on a task makes us feel good. When we manage to shut out distraction and calm our minds, we can fully enjoy the task at hand. We also need concentration in order to think more deeply about a situation or process intellectually.

- Get a pen and a piece of paper and just doodle. Studies from Harvard Health show that doodling helps keep the mind focused, especially when we have to listen and absorb information over a longer period of time. Doodling or free drawing also relieves stress and gives an insight into our emotional state.

- While there seems to be no way to completely stop our drunken monkeys, we can tame them and live with them better. Meditation yoga and other disciplines help. And of course Sophrology! Sophrology has a set of exercises for concentrating the mind and helping it work as efficiently as possible. To do anything successfully in life, and we include doing nothing in that, it helps to concentrate. Let these exercises aid you in doing just that.

Setting Intentions

Reflect on and write down situations where you want to concentrate and focus:

- _____
- _____
- _____

As you do the exercises keep these situations in mind.

The Third Eye

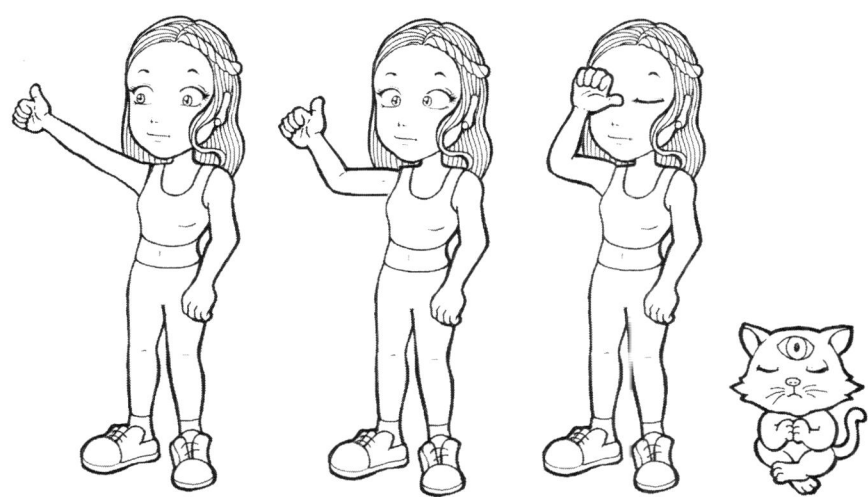

Stand up.

Keep your eyes open.

Raise your right arm to the horizontal level.

Close your hand to make a fist and point your thumb towards the sky, as if you were hitch-hiking.

Breathe in deeply through your nose and hold your breath.

Slowly bring your thumb back towards your forehead while staring at it intently.

Let your thumb touch the point between your eyes.

Imagine planting concentration in your head as you close your eyes.

Breathe out through your mouth and relax your arm by your side.

Breathe naturally again.

Notice your sensations.

Feel the sensations in your forehead and eyes.

Become aware of the point between your eyes.

Open your eyes and do the exercise a second time.

Raise your right arm to the horizontal level.

Close your hand to make a fist and point your thumb towards the sky, as if you were hitch-hiking.

Breathe in deeply through your nose and hold your breath.

Slowly bring your thumb back towards your forehead while staring at it intently.

Let your thumb touch the point between your eyes.

Imagine installing concentration in your head as you close your eyes.

Breathe out through your mouth and relax your arm by your side.

Breathe naturally again.

Notice your sensations.

Think about the point between your eyes.

Become aware of your powers of concentration

Open your eyes and do the exercise a third time.

Raise your right arm to the horizontal level.

Close your hand to make a fist and point your thumb towards the sky, as if you were hitch-hiking.

Breathe in deeply through your nose and hold your breath.

Slowly bring your thumb back towards your forehead while staring at it intently.

Let your thumb touch the point between your eyes.

Imagine your mind fully concentrating as you close your eyes.

Breathe out through your mouth and relax your arm by your side.

Breathe naturally again.

Notice your sensations.

Welcome all your feelings.

Become aware of your capacity to concentrate.

The exercise is now finished and you can open your eyes.

Object Concentration

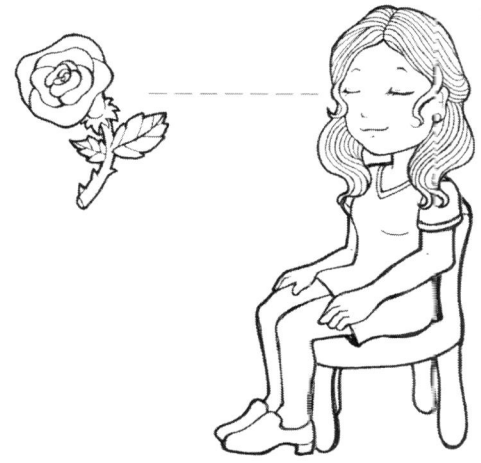

Sit down.

Close your eyes.

Allow the image of an object to come into your head.

Concentrate on this object.

Imagine its physical properties.

Observe its shape.

Imagine its colours and brightness.

Take in what it's made of.

Welcome all the feelings that you experience.

Observe the object from every angle.

Give it all of your attention.

Notice your sensations.

Welcome all your feelings.

Become aware of your capacity to concentrate.

The exercise is now finished and you can open your eyes.

Come To Your Senses

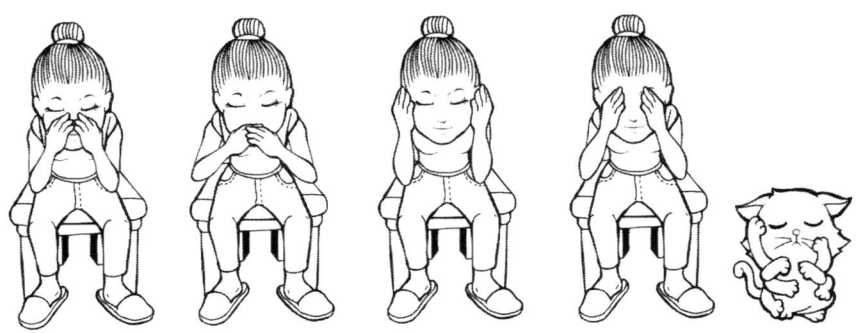

Sit down.

Close your eyes.

Touch

Think about your sense of touch.

Touch your head and face.

Imagine their shape and texture.

Touch your neck.

Feel the difference in sensations between your skin and your clothes.

Go down your body with your fingers.

Touch your arms, your chest, your stomach, your legs, your feet.

Slowly sit up straight again and put your hands on your thighs.

Imagine feeling some lovely textures and materials.

Become aware of your fingers and of the sense of touch.

Feel how your sense of touch connects you with the world.

Smell

Think about your nose.

Touch it and rediscover its shape.

Touch your nostrils.

Feel the fresh air as you inhale.

Feel the warmer air as you exhale.

Put your hands on your thighs again.

Breathe in the smells around you.

Imagine some pleasant aromas.

Become aware of your nose and of the sense of smell.

Feel how your sense of smell connects you with the world.

Taste

Think about your mouth.

Touch your lips and feel their shape.

Become aware of your tongue and pallet.

Pass your tongue over your teeth.

Taste your saliva.

Put your hands on your thighs again.

Imagine some gorgeous tastes.

Become aware of your mouth and of the sense of taste.

Feel how your sense of taste connects you with the world.

Hearing

Think about your ears.

Put your elbows on your knees and touch your ears.

Put the palms of your hands over your ears and vary the intensity of the pressure.

Hear the different noises.

Put your hands on your thighs again.

Imagine hearing some beautiful melodies and exquisite sounds.

Become aware of your ears and of the sense of hearing.

Feel how your sense of hearing connects you with the world.

Sight

Bring your attention to your eyes.

Touch your eyelashes and eyelids.

Feel your eyeballs as they move around.

Put your fingers on your eyelids and move them around slowly and gently.

See the different colours and luminosities.

Put your hands on your thighs again.

Picture some stunning and beautiful landscapes.

Become aware of your eyes and of the sense of sight.

Feel how your sense of sight connects you with the world.

Treasure and value all the senses that you have.

Feel your connection with the world.

The exercise is now finished and you can open your eyes.

Chapter 5: BOOST YOUR CONFIDENCE

So you think you lack confidence in something, or in general. So what? We all do. There are many reasons why we might lack confidence. It could be our upbringing or a toxic person in our lives. Or simply because we are new to something and haven't got any experience in it yet. Once you've scanned your life for what could be munching away at your confidence and hopefully kicked it out, you can then start to build up what you think you might be lacking, whether it is a certain skill or just how you see yourself.

We want to show you some useful tricks that enable us to feel more confident immediately and build this confidence up more permanently.

But first what to do when the doubts set in? Ah - the questions surrounding the big "What if?"… What if I am not good enough? What if I can't convince? What if I get nervous? We've all gone through similar questions. But what is the worst thing that could happen? If we are honest, in most cases nothing much! Furthermore, who decides if we are good enough? Do we need to convince everybody? And doesn't being nervous sometimes make us appear more human and likeable? The answer to the scary "What if?" questions is often "So What!"

- We become confident by putting our abilities and skills to the test. For that we need to overcome our inhibitions and work up the courage to step out of our comfort zone. Just like a young bird needs to step out of its nest in order to learn to fly. One step towards the goal of improving our confidence is to always see ourselves in a process of development. In this way we allow ourselves to take more risks and make mistakes.

- Another step is to think and talk well about ourselves and to ourselves. Don't put yourself down, especially in front of others. Be very careful with self-deprecating humour. Unless you're a professional comedian who gets paid for it!

- Another tip is to practise Power Poses. Give it a try! Do the Superman! Stand with your legs apart, hold your head up high and stretch your arm to the sky for a couple of minutes! But be careful not to take off! Or do a Wonder Woman with legs apart and hands on your hips.

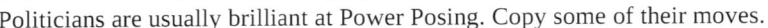

There are many studies to prove that these poses send empowering messages to the brain and therefore help with building up confidence. Politicians are usually brilliant at Power Posing. Copy some of their moves.

- Don't listen to other people's opinion. Or, if we need an opinion just choose a few people we find trustworthy and helpful. And just flush the rest down the mental toilet.

- And remind yourself of your successes. Sometimes we forget that we have already succeeded in many things. We once had to learn and become good at the things that seem normal to us now. But that's why we have a best friend in Sophrology, to remind us to count our past successes and be proud.

So once you have done all the above, try the following combination of exercises to really anchor this confidence stuff in your everyday life.

The "No" and "Yes" exercises are designed to help us easily say these words, which some of us find difficult under pressure.

Note: There's nothing wrong with giving a "Definitely Maybe" response to a question. Except that sometimes we only do this to avoid the inevitable "No" answer which we will have to give at some point!

The visualization exercise "Personal Gesture" helps give us a boost when we need it.

"Pride From My Past" aims to give us more confidence as we look at the positive things we've achieved in our lives.

If we're doing something new, it's completely normal not to feel confident. But we shouldn't let it affect our wider opinion of ourselves.

Setting Intentions

With the following exercises we aim to increase your overall confidence. The idea is to strengthen your ability to say "No" when you want to. And to stick to the "No"! And conversely to say "Yes" to opportunities, especially if you feel you have missed some in the past! We will also help you anchor a positive emotion with a gesture that you can call upon when you need it. And we will help you remember all the things you have accomplished in the past so you can be proud of your achievements!

You may notice that each exercise has a different intention. To help you, we have added intention boxes.

The "No" Exercise

Setting Intentions

Reflect on and write down situations where you want to say "No" and the reasons why:

- _____
- _____
- _____

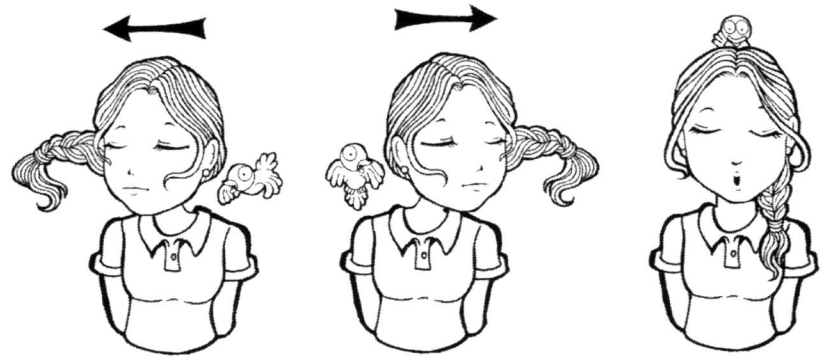

Stand up.

Close your eyes.

Breathe in through your nose and hold your breath.

Slowly turn your head from left to right as if you were saying "No".

Imagine saying "No" to things that are not in your best interests.

Breathe out through your mouth while bringing your head back to its starting position.

Breathe naturally again.

Notice your sensations.

Feel the movement in your neck

Become aware of the relaxation in your neck.

Do the exercise a second time.

Breathe in through your nose and hold your breath.

Slowly turn your head from left to right as if you were saying "No".

Imagine saying "No" to things that you don't want to do.

Breathe out through your mouth while bringing your head back to its starting position.

Breathe naturally again.

Notice your sensations.

Think about the distance your head moved.

Become aware of your capacity to refuse something that goes against your will.

Do the exercise a third time.

Breathe in through your nose and hold your breath.

Slowly turn your head from left to right as if you were saying "No".

Imagine being able to say "No" whenever you want to.

Breathe out through your mouth while bringing your head back to its starting position.

Breathe naturally again.

Notice your sensations.

Welcome all your feelings.

Become aware of your capacity to say "No".

The exercise is now finished and you can open your eyes.

The "Yes" Exercise

Setting Intentions

Reflect on and write down situations/opportunities where you want to say "Yes" and the reasons why:

- _____
- _____
- _____

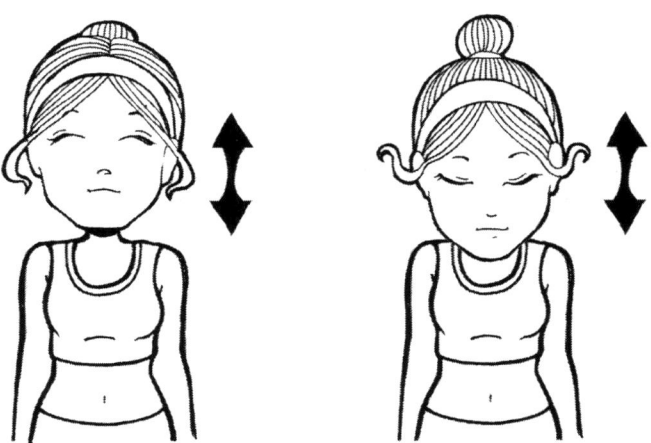

Stand up.

Close your eyes.

Breathe in through your nose and hold your breath.

Slowly move your head up and down as if you were saying "Yes".

Imagine saying "Yes" to things that are in your best interests.

Breathe out through your mouth while bringing your head back to its starting position.

Breathe naturally again.

Notice your sensations.

Feel the movement in your neck.

Become aware of the relaxation in your neck.

Do the exercise a second time.

Breathe in through your nose and hold your breath.

Slowly move your head up and down as if you were saying "Yes".

Imagine saying "Yes" to things that you want to do.

Breathe out through your mouth while bringing your head back to its starting position.

Breathe naturally again.

Notice your sensations.

Think about the distance your head moved.

Become aware of your capacity to say "Yes" to opportunities.

Do the exercise a third time.

Breathe in through your nose and hold your breath.

Slowly move your head up and down as if you were saying "Yes".

Imagine being able to say "Yes" whenever you want to.

Breathe out through your mouth while bringing your head back to its starting position.

Breathe naturally again.

Notice your sensations.

Welcome all your feelings.

Become aware of your capacity to say "Yes".

The exercise is now finished and you can open your eyes.

Personal Gesture

Setting Intentions

Write down a great moment/event from your life that comes into your mind:

- _____

The idea of this exercise is to anchor positive feelings with a personal gesture. Ideally this is a gesture that nobody else will notice. Some examples include:

- Holding the wrist of one arm with the hand of the other.
- Touching your thumb and one of your fingers.
- Holding hands with yourself.

Feel free to choose whatever gesture is comfortable for you!

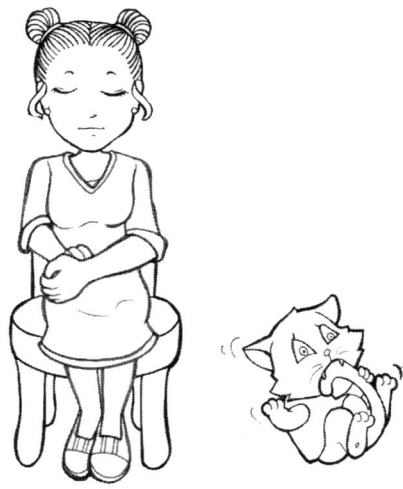

Sit down.

Close your eyes.

Remember a really positive event in your life.

A moment when you were fully yourself.

A moment of great happiness.

Take the time to relive the scene

What did you see, hear, smell and feel?

Picture the scene in your mind.

The people who surrounded you, the place where you were, all the different objects.

Relive the sounds that you heard.

Breathe in the smells and touch the objects all around you.

Fully relive the moment.

Now anchor this moment with your personal gesture.

Really be aware of all the sensations in your body.

Are they the same everywhere?

Are they stronger in some parts of your body than in others?

Note your feelings as you relive this fantastic moment.

Become aware of all your sensations.

Hold the physical gesture for as long as you like.

When you're ready, release the gesture and return to your normal seated position.

Feel the confidence inside your body.

Remember that these sensations are always present in you.

Think about them in your daily life when you want to feel confident.

Use your personal gesture to bring back these positive sensations when you need or want them.

The exercise is now finished and you can open your eyes.

Pride From My Past

Setting Intentions

Reflect on and write down some of the greatest moments of your life (write down more than three if you want):

- _____
- _____
- _____

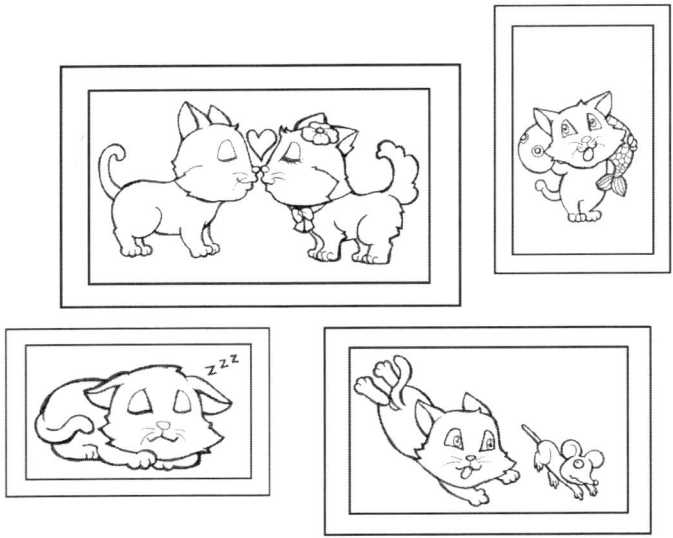

Sit down.

Close your eyes.

Go through your life and remember some of the great moments.

Bring back all your joy and happiness.

Welcome all these memories into your mind.

Don't hold back, let them flood in.

Fully relive the great moments from your life.

Savour the feelings that you have on remembering these events.

Take the time to fully explore them and look at them in detail.

Make a photo album of the highlights of your life.

Appreciate all their beneficial effects.

Really feel the positive sensations that life can bring you.

Remember that these sensations are always present in you.

Think about them in your daily life when you want to feel confident.

The exercise is now finished and you can open your eyes.

Chapter 6: BOOST YOUR ENERGY

It's great to wake up in the morning, really looking forward to what the day will bring! To be curious and full of energy! To shoot out of bed like a cannonball!

That being said, we don't always feel as energetic as we'd like to.

There are many reasons we could be lacking energy to do the things that we want to do. We've already looked at some of them in this book, for example feeling stressed.

How much energy we have available depends to some extent on how much we "waste" on these "negative" activities. Sophrology helps us remove blockages and focus on the tasks that are most important to us.

But maybe you just need a little energy boost. If so, this chapter is for you!

● Feel the energy stored in your body as you "Walk on the Spot", start releasing it with the "Shoulder Pump" and fully feel your vitality with the "Jumping Jack" exercise. Then visualize yourself in nature, renewing your energy and recharging your batteries next to a waterfall. Finally, fill yourself up with energy on a sophrological "Trip to the Sun".

Nature is a good place to see energy and vitality at work. "Nature does not hurry, yet everything is accomplished," said Lao Tzu.

Setting Intentions

Reflect on and write down the areas in your life that you would like to energize or revitalize:

- _____
- _____
- _____

Walk On The Spot

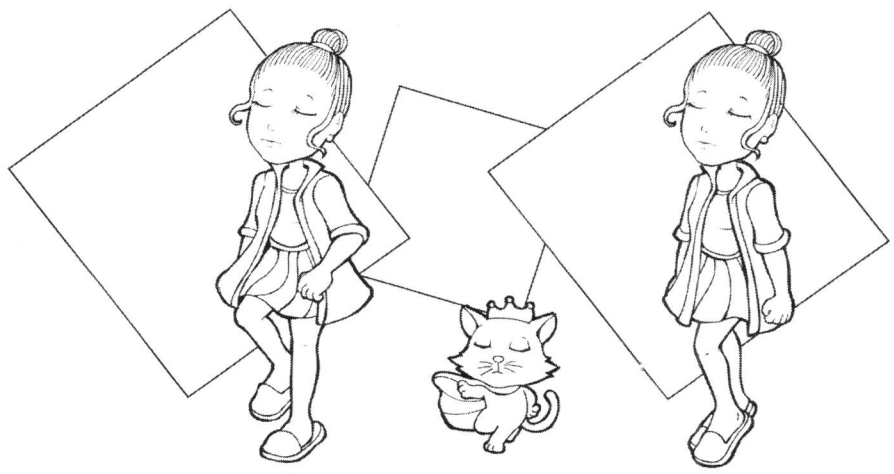

Stand up.

Close your eyes.

Walk slowly on the spot while breathing normally.

Break down your steps into their component parts.

Imagine them in detail in your mind's eye.

Feel the transfer of energy from one side of your body to the other.

Feel the power of your muscles.

Imagine the power stored in your body.

Stop when you wish.

Notice your sensations.

Feel the sensations in your legs and feet.

Become aware of your balance.

Do the exercise a second time.

Walk slowly on the spot.

Break down your steps into their component parts.

Imagine them in detail in your mind's eye.

Feel the transfer of power from one side of your body to the other.

Feel the energy that goes into each movement.

Imagine the energy stored in your body.

Stop when you wish.

Notice your sensations.

Feel the balance between the two sides of your body.

Become aware of the energy stored in your body.

Do the exercise a third time.

Walk slowly on the spot.

Break down your steps into their component parts.

Imagine them in detail in your mind's eye.

Feel the transfer of energy and power from one side of your body to the other.

Feel the energy you're putting into the world with each step.

Imagine advancing towards your goals, full of energy.

Stop when you wish.

Notice your sensations.

Welcome all your feelings.

Become aware of your capacity to walk towards your goals full of energy.

The exercise is now finished and you can open your eyes.

Shoulder Pump

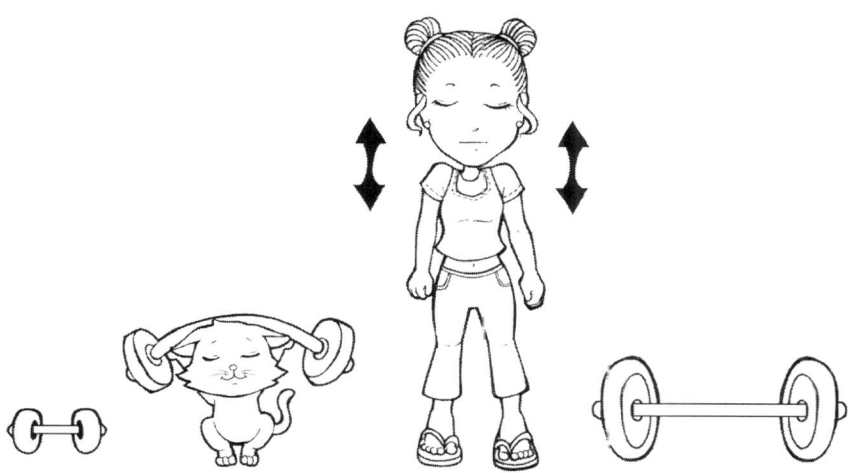

Stand up.

Shut your eyes.

Close your hands and make them into fists.

Breathe in through your nose and hold your breath.

Move your shoulders up and down a number of times.

Imagine the energy flowing through you with each pump.

Exhale strongly through your mouth as you relax your shoulders and open up your hands.

Breathe naturally again.

Notice your sensations.

Welcome all the sensations in your shoulders, arms and hands.

Become aware of the relaxation of your shoulders, arms and hands.

Do the exercise a second time.

Close your hands and make them into fists.

Breathe in through your nose and hold your breath.

Move your shoulders up and down a number of times.

Imagine increasing your energy with each pump.

Exhale strongly through your mouth as you relax your shoulders and open up your hands.

Breathe naturally again.

Notice your sensations.

Welcome the feelings in your shoulders and chest.

Become aware that your body is full of energy.

Do the exercise a third time.

Close your hands and make them into fists.

Breathe in through your nose and hold your breath.

Move your shoulders up and down a number of times.

Imagine increasing your vitality with each pump.

Exhale strongly through your mouth as you relax your shoulders and open up your hands.

Breathe naturally again.

Notice your sensations.

Welcome all your feelings.

Become aware of your capacity to increase your vitality.

The exercise is now finished and you can open your eyes.

Jumping Jack

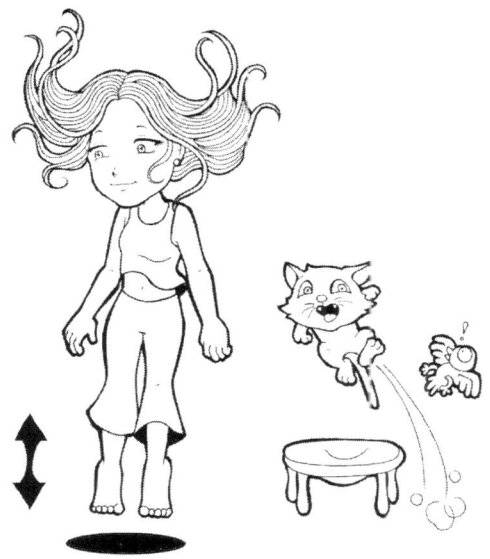

Stand up.

Keep your eyes open.

Jump up and down while breathing naturally.

Relax your arms and head as you jump.

You can really let go!

Imagine all the energy inside you.

Imagine increasing your energy with each jump.

Continue for as long as you like.

Stop when you've had enough.

Close your eyes.

Notice your sensations.

Welcome all your feelings.

Become aware and feel the energy inside you.

The exercise is now finished and you can open your eyes.

Waterfall Visualization

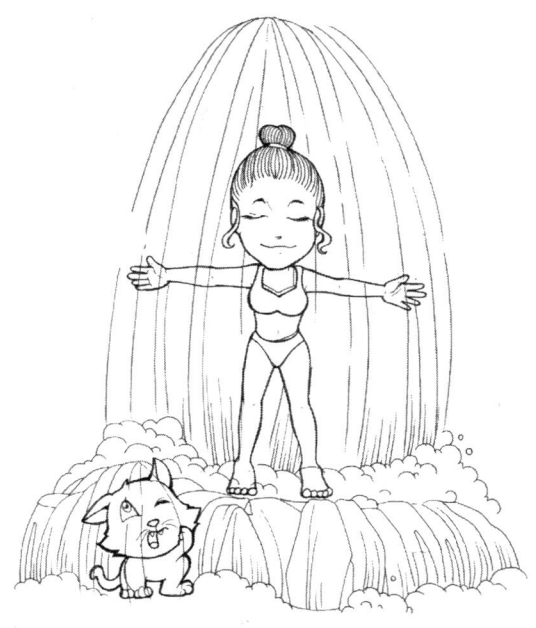

Sit down.

Close your eyes.

Imagine yourself near a beautiful, natural waterfall.

Let the image of it come into your mind.

Imagine the waterfall in great detail.

See the landscape all around it.

Watch the clean, fresh water head off towards its destination, full of energy and power.

Become aware that nothing will stop the water from reaching its goal.

Bring your attention to the sounds that surround you.

Hear the water descend from a great height.

Become aware of the energy that is released as the water falls.

Touch the water.

Feel it flow through your hands.

Go and stand under the waterfall.

Feel the energy of the water on your body.

Taste the clean, fresh water.

Feel this source of life giving you energy.

Welcome all the positive sensations that this image gives you.

Become aware of all these sensations in your body.

Spread them throughout your body.

Remember that these sensations are always present in you.

Think about them in your daily life when you need a boost of energy.

The exercise is now finished and you can open your eyes.

Trip To The Sun

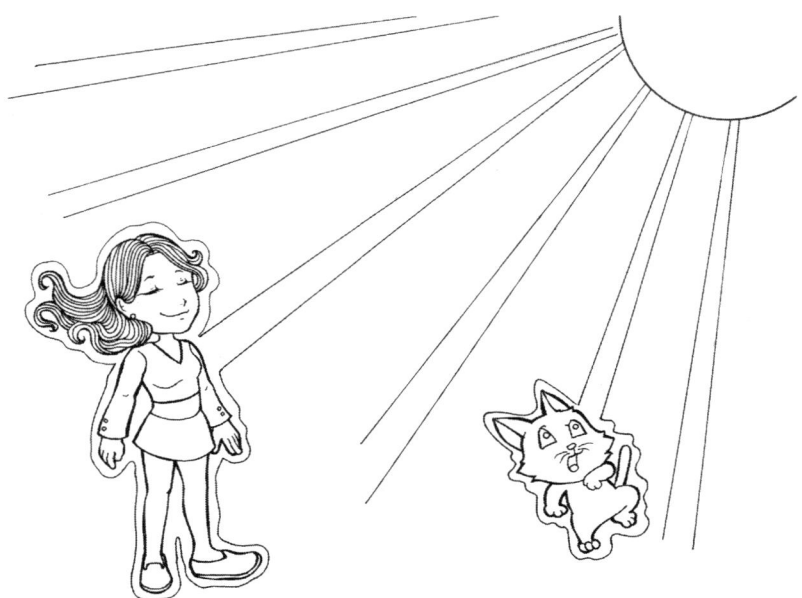

Sit down.

Close your eyes.

Imagine your body.

Picture it where you are right now.

Now look down on it from above.

See yourself in your surroundings.

Continue to look at your body from above, but now go higher and higher.

See the place where you live.

Imagine your town and region.

Picture your country with its borders.

Think about the continents and the seas.

Continue your ascension so you can see the whole of the Earth.

Now go on a sophrological trip towards the Sun.

You pass the Moon.

You see Venus and Mercury.

And now you are approaching your destination.

As this is a sophrological trip, the Sun is of no danger to you.

You start orbiting around the Sun, taking in the energy that it is emitting.

The Sun lights up your body, lights up your personality.

You are glowing with energy inside and outside.

You can get as close as you want to the Sun and even go inside it without any risk.

You dive into the Sun and bathe in its source of intense energy.

It charges you up and fills you with vitality and strength.

Before you leave the Sun you consciously take in all the cosmic energy you can.

You are aware that this source of energy is always available to you when you need it.

This well of energy is forever there for you.

Prepare yourself to slowly make your return trip to Earth.

You go past Mercury and Venus.

You see the beauty of our planet from space as you fly past the Moon.

You begin your descent.

Picture the continents and the oceans.

See your country with its borders and features.

Slowly continue your descent.

Visualize your region.

Pick out the place where you are.

Look down on your body from above.

Observe its inner energy and vitality.

Know that every time you take in the Sun's rays, they are filling you with energy, strength and light.

Spread these sensations throughout your body.

Remember that these sensations are always present in you.

Think about them in your daily life when you need a boost of energy.

The exercise is now finished and you can open your eyes.

Chapter 7: SHINE AT ANY EVENT

This chapter focuses on preparing for an important event. For example a business meeting, a job interview, a sports match, giving birth or an exam. Please keep in mind that having goals and objectives about the outcome of any event contributes largely to its success.

Sophrology helps in two main ways:

- Keeping us relaxed before and during the event.

It's not just the occasion itself that's important. It's how we live the days and hours before it that will go a long way to determine whether it's a success for us.

If we're overstressed beforehand, we will not only damage our lives in the lead-up to The Big Day, but we're also far less likely to perform at our best. (That's why it's important to prepare with some of the exercises from the previous chapters.)

- Helping us visualize the day of the event in detail, before it happens.

If we haven't visualized everything that could happen, the smallest problem might throw us. To be clear, in order to feel confident, we need to believe we will do well. That is the purpose of the first visualization, which delights in our feelings after a successful event.

But Sophrology does not brush the potential or real problems under the carpet. The more we have visualized what to do when things don't go perfectly, the better prepared we will be for every eventuality. The second visualization looks at the whole day of the event, from the moment we wake up until it's finished. The idea is to imagine everything that can go right or wrong. Go through each moment so that we're ready for it all.

Of course, all the visualization in the world won't help if we haven't put in the work as well. To take an obvious example, imagine wanting to run a marathon and only doing relaxation and visualization exercises! Sophrology is a great accompaniment for our big event preparations, but it doesn't substitute for the preparations themselves!

But put the two together and it's amazing how strong we can be!

Pre-Live Your Future Success

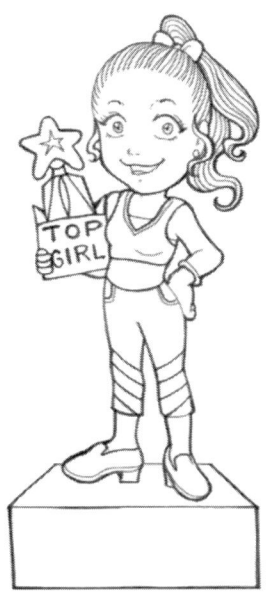

Part 1 - After The Event

Sit down.

Close your eyes.

You have just finished the event that you have been preparing for.

After all your hard work, the event has been a great success.

This is a really fantastic moment for you.

Take the time to imagine the scene.

What do you see, hear, smell and feel?

Picture everything in your mind.

Imagine where you are and the smiles of those around you.

Pay attention to the sounds that you hear.

The talking and the laughing.

The congratulations you receive.

Breathe in the smells. The smells of success.

Fully live this moment.

Feel the relief of having accomplished what you set out to do.

The pride in your achievement.

Experience the joy that you feel on having reached your objective.

The satisfaction of having given the best of yourself.

Savour your triumph.

Be fully aware of all the physical, mental and emotional sensations in your body.

Let these wonderful sensations flow right through you.

Notice the positive feelings throughout your body.

Remember that these sensations are always present in you.

Think about them on the day of your big event.

The exercise is now finished and you can open your eyes.

Part 2 - The Day Of The Event

Note: Naturally the details of the day will be different depending on what the big event is (making a speech, passing an exam, giving birth etc.) The example given below is thus somewhat generic. You can change the details to suit your event.

Sit down.

Close your eyes.

Imagine yourself on the day of your big event.

You wake up in the morning.

You are ready for the day ahead.

Take the time to imagine what you see, hear, smell and feel.

Picture the scene in your mind.

You follow your daily morning routine.

Maybe you wash, eat and drink something.

You get dressed in the clothes that you will be wearing for the day.

Pause a moment to become aware of your feelings.

Maybe some excitement about what is to come. Maybe some fear too.

Be aware of all the physical, mental and emotional sensations linked to your big day.

You go to where the event will be happening.

Picture the scene in your mind.

The people and the place, the different objects that surround you.

Imagine the event beginning.

You are doing all the things you have been preparing for.

Perhaps there are some difficulties and unexpected problems.

You find solutions for these simply and easily.

Maybe you will be able to come back later to those you can't solve at the time.

Pay attention to all the sounds that you hear.

The talking and the laughter that are around you.

Breathe in the smells.

Touch an object that's close to you.

Appreciate that you are giving the best of yourself.

Feel the pride of living out the moment you have been preparing for.

Become aware of all your physical, mental and emotional sensations as you experience your big event.

You have now finished the event.

After all your hard work, it has been a great success.

This is a really fantastic moment for you.

Take the time to imagine the scene.

What do you see, hear, smell and feel?

Picture the scene in your mind.

Pay attention to the sounds that you hear.

The talking and the laughing.

The congratulations you receive.

Breathe in the smells.

Fully live this moment of great personal success.

Feel the relief of having accomplished what you set out to do.

Feel the pride in your achievement.

Experience the joy of having reached your objective.

The satisfaction of having given the best of yourself.

Savour your triumph.

Be fully aware of all the physical, mental and emotional sensations in your body.

Let these wonderful sensations flow right through you.

Notice the positive feelings throughout your body.

Remember that these sensations are always present in you.

Think about them on the day of your big event.

The exercise is now finished and you can open your eyes.

Chapter 8: FEEL THE NEW YOU

Life is always changing and change happens whether we like it or not. As Robert C. Gallagher said, "Change is inevitable. Except from a vending machine."

The basic idea of this final chapter is to recognise our progress. It's intended to be positive and encouraging.

Some changes are desired and chances are, if you are reading this little guide, that you are actively and intentionally seeking them. You are taking charge to figure out what you need in order to get it. That takes a lot of courage. This means you are willing to change the way you see yourself and implement it in your life. Our brains like to resist that kind of change. For example, imagine the devoted wife who finally admits to feeling suffocated in her marriage and asks for a divorce or the person in a boring and dead-end job who attempts to strike out in a new direction. Or maybe it's about something subtler, like learning a new skill or being more assertive, etc. Whether we want to change something big or small, it is brave.

And then sometimes, as part of this natural process of change, it's good to stop and take stock of what we've done and how far we've come.

In the Relaxed Movement exercises you'll become aware of all parts of your body. If you've made changes recently, these can often be felt physically. Do you feel more solid, more present, more you?

This chapter contains two visualization exercises. First you hold up a "Sophro Mirror" to yourself to become aware of the new you. Second you project yourself into the future and explain to a loved one how you overcame the problem you were working on. This exercise is called "Back to the Future".

Becoming aware of how much we've developed is another important role our best friends can play for us. Sometimes we can't see it ourselves. Besties can show us how far we've advanced, when we forget.

Setting Intentions

Reflect on and write down the different ways you have changed recently!

- _____
- _____
- _____

Keep these changes in mind when you do the exercises!

Feel Your Head

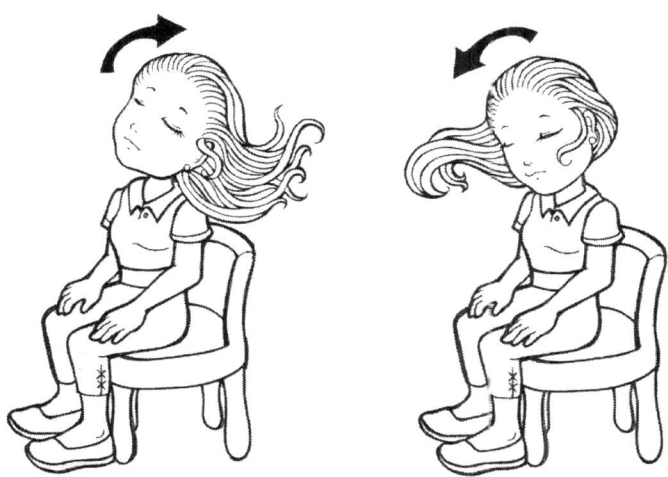

Sit down.

Close your eyes.

Lean your head slightly backwards.

Breathe in through your nose and hold your breath.

Imagine your head as the command centre of your body.

Slowly bring your head back to its normal position while breathing out through your mouth.

Breathe naturally again.

Notice your sensations.

Feel the volume of your head.

Become aware of the density of your head.

Do the exercise a second time with your head leaning slightly forwards.

Lean your head slightly forwards.

Breathe in through your nose and hold your breath.

Imagine your head as the house of your eyes, ears, nose and mouth.

Slowly bring your head back to its normal position while breathing out through your mouth.

Breathe naturally again.

Notice your sensations.

Feel the weight of your head.

Become aware that your head houses four of your senses.

Do the exercise a third time, choosing the starting position of your head.

Lean your head slightly forwards or backwards.

Breathe in through your nose and hold your breath.

Imagine your head as the house of your brain.

Slowly bring your head back to its normal position while breathing out through your mouth.

Breathe naturally again.

Notice your sensations.

Welcome all your feelings.

Become fully conscious of the mental, emotional and physical importance of your head.

The exercise is now finished and you can open your eyes.

Feel Your Arms

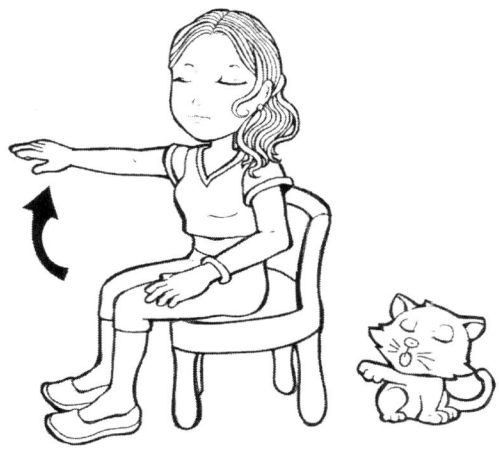

Sit down.

Close your eyes.

Lift your right arm up to the horizontal position.

Breathe in through your nose and hold your breath.

Imagine taking what you need from the physical world.

Slowly lower your arm and place your hand on your thigh while breathing out through your mouth.

Breathe naturally again.

Notice your sensations.

Feel the volume of your right arm.

Become aware of the strength of your arm.

Do the exercise a second time using your left arm.

Lift your left arm up to the horizontal position.

Breathe in through your nose and hold your breath.

Imagine giving what you want to the physical world.

Slowly lower your arm and place your hand on your thigh while breathing out through your mouth.

Breathe naturally again.

Notice your sensations.

Feel the density of your left arm.

Become aware of the power of your arm.

Do the exercise a third time using both your arms.

Lift both arms up to the horizontal position.

Breathe in through your nose and hold your breath.

Imagine your arms creating and changing the material world.

Slowly lower your arms and place your hands on your thighs while breathing out through your mouth.

Breathe naturally again.

Notice your sensations.

Welcome all your feelings.

Become fully conscious of the strength and power of your arms.

The exercise is now finished and you can open your eyes.

Feel Your Legs

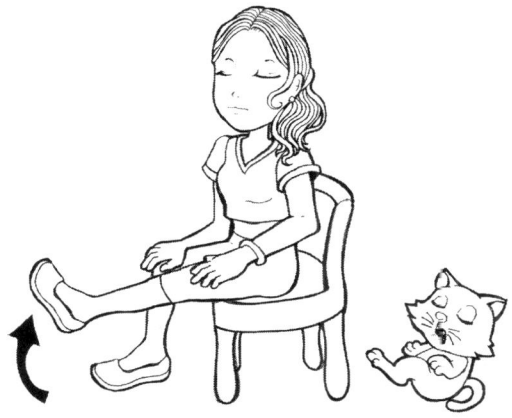

Sit down.

Close your eyes.

Lift your right leg up to the horizontal position.

Breathe in through your nose and hold your breath.

Imagine moving towards your goals at your own pace.

Slowly lower your leg while breathing out through your mouth.

Breathe naturally again.

Notice your sensations.

Feel the volume of your right leg.

Become aware of the strength of your leg.

Do the exercise a second time, using your left leg.

Lift your left leg up to the horizontal position.

Breathe in through your nose and hold your breath.

Imagine moving firmly and solidly towards your goals.

Slowly lower your leg while breathing out through your mouth.

Breathe naturally again.

Notice your sensations.

Feel the density of your left leg.

Become aware of the power of your leg.

Do the exercise a third time using both your legs.

Lift both legs up to the horizontal position.

Breathe in through your nose and hold your breath.

Imagine using your legs to move firmly towards your goals.

Slowly lower your legs while breathing out through your mouth.

Breathe naturally again.

Notice your sensations.

Welcome all your feelings.

Become fully conscious of the strength and power of your legs.

The exercise is now finished and you can open your eyes.

Feel Your Body

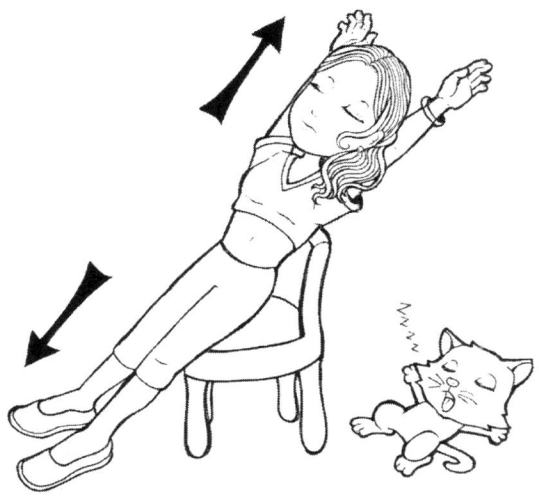

Sit down.

Close your eyes.

Raise your arms above your head and lift up your legs.

Breathe in through your nose and hold your breath.

Gently stretch your body.

Imagine being fully conscious of your body in the here and now.

Appreciate your place in space and time.

Return to the starting position while breathing out through your mouth.

Breathe naturally again.

Notice your sensations.

Feel the volume of your body.

Become aware of the strength of your body.

Do the exercise a second time.

Raise your arms above your head and lift up your legs.

Breathe in through your nose and hold your breath.

Gently stretch your body.

Imagine being fully conscious of the strength of your body.

Appreciate the power of your body as it interacts with the world.

Return to the starting position while breathing out through your mouth.

Breathe naturally again.

Notice your sensations.

Feel the density of your body.

Become aware of the strength of your body.

Do the exercise a third time.

Raise your arms above your head and lift up your legs.

Breathe in through your nose and hold your breath.

Gently stretch your body.

Imagine being fully conscious of your body from your head to your toes.

Appreciate the unique features that make you who you are.

Return to the starting position while breathing out through your mouth.

Breathe naturally again.

Notice your sensations.

Welcome all your feelings.

Become fully conscious of your body.

The exercise is now finished and you can open your eyes.

Sophro Mirror

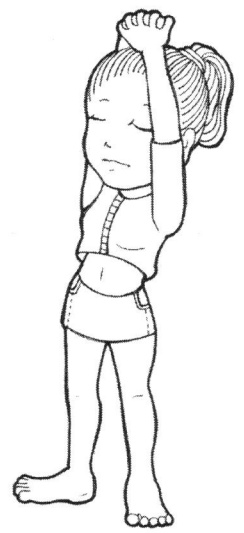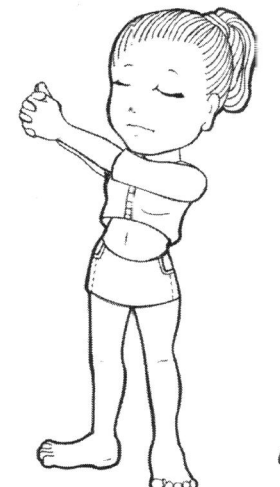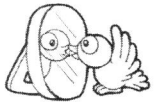

Stand up.

Close your eyes.

Join your hands together and lift them above your head.

Slowly bring your hands down in front of your body.

Imagine your palms are a mirror.

Project the image of your body in the palms of your hands.

See the image of your brain, your eyes, your nose, your ears, your mouth.

Notice how you feel, looking at them from the outside.

Continue to lower your hands at your own speed.

Observe your chest and stomach which are rising and falling with each breath.

Project the image of your waist, hips and sexual organs.

Now look at your legs and feet.

Continue to lower your hands at your own speed until you've observed your whole body, from head to toe.

Slowly stand up again.

Notice your sensations.

Welcome all your feelings.

Become aware of how you see the new you.

Think about how it compares to an earlier you.

The exercise is now finished and you can open your eyes.

Back To The Future

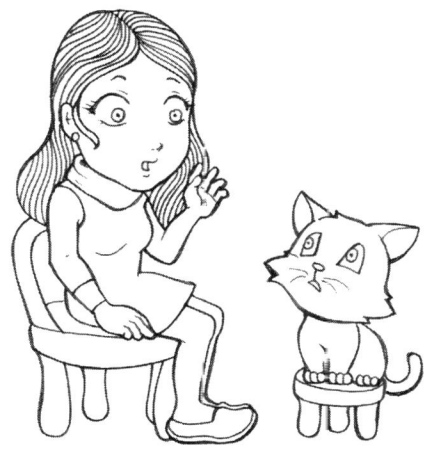

Sit down.

Close your eyes.

Imagine yourself in the future.

You are talking to a close friend about a problem that you have overcome.

Take the time to imagine the scene with your friend.

What do you see, hear, smell and feel?

Hear yourself talking about the difficulties that you overcame.

Explain the fears and worries that you had.

Talk about how you wondered if you would ever overcome the problem.

Admit that you had doubts.

Now explain to your friend exactly how you succeeded.

How little by little you understood how to solve the problem.

Talk about what you did in order to go past the problem.

The path you took to overcome your difficulties.

Explain the difference between your fears and the reality.

Talk about how it was easier than you imagined.

Go into all the emotions you felt after your victory.

Spread these sensations throughout your body.

Remember that these sensations are always present in you.

Think about them in your daily life when you want to recognise your potential.

The exercise is now finished and you can open your eyes.

THE THREE TECHNIQUES

Sophrology uses three means to achieve its aims of increasing our consciousness. They are:

- Controlled Breathing
- Relaxed Movement exercises
- Visualization

Let's look briefly at all three.

Controlled Breathing

One controlled breathing technique is repeated very often in this book. The idea is to breathe in and hold your breath while doing a Relaxed Movement exercise.

This has the effect of concentrating our minds on what we're doing and heightening our awareness of what we're feeling.

The idea of Sophrology is to increase our conscicusness and the controlled breathing helps achieve that aim.

There are two other breathing techniques that you will also find in the exercises.

- Breathe in and put a positive thought in your head. Breathe out to spread this idea throughout your body. Try it now! With calmness for example. Breathe in calmness and fix the idea in your head. Breathe out and diffuse it throughout your body.

- Breathe in something positive like calmness, breathe out something negative like stress. Or as one wag put it, "Breathe in the good shit. Breathe out the bullshit."

Note: Sophrology encourages the slow, deep abdominal breathing that we naturally do when we sleep.

Relaxed Movement Exercises

We all have experience of being mentally stressed and also feeling physically tense in different parts of our bodies. Usually if we manage to de-stress our minds, our bodies will follow suit. This can be done by meditating or breathing deeply for example. Of course, there are other ways but we recommend these two!

Edmund Jacobson (1888 - 1983) postulated that the reverse could happen too. In other words, if we relax our body, we will feel less stressed in our minds. This somewhat revolutionary idea at the time has become common knowledge since. We all know that exercise can relax us.

The Relaxed Movement exercises that you find in this book can be used as simple stress relievers. But to Alfonso Caycedo they were so much more. Caycedo used them as a means to increase our awareness and help us more generally in life. And one of the ways he did that was by combining them with visualization exercises. Which is our next section!

Visualization

Visualization is an incredibly powerful tool. The Swiss ski team in the 1960's were one of the first to use Sophrology's visualization exercises. They had a huge success at the 1968 Winter Olympics which really gave the new discipline of Sophrology a public boost at the time.

Caycedo later worked with champion golfer Severiano Ballesteros, who attributed a lot of his success to Sophrology. He said, "I practised Sophrology and I firmly believe that I owe my success to it."

We're all champions in a way! And visualization helps us as much as it helps well-known people.

It has been proven that real-life events and their imagined counterparts have a similar effect on the brain. Meaning that the brain sends the same messages to the body and nervous system if an event is real or imagined. Caycedo knew how to use this fact to create Sophrology's visualization exercises, some of which you'll find in this book. We hope you gain as much from them as we have!

About The Founder: ALFONSO CAYCEDO

What do you do if you're a doctor in a field (neuropsychiatry) and you don't like what your speciality offers your patients? If your name's Alfonso Caycedo, you decide to spend the rest of your life creating a new discipline that works better. He was looking for less invasive treatments and wanted a more holistic approach.

But before he could create he needed to discover. Caycedo (1932 - 2017) spent time in countries like Switzerland, India and Japan and worked with experts including the 14th Dalai Lama and Ludwig Binswanger, the founder of phenomenological psychology.

In 1960 he invented the name Sophrology which is made up of three parts that come from Greek:

Sos: Harmony

Phren: Spirit or consciousness

Logos: Science or study

Sophrology means the study of consciousness in harmony.

This beautifully pieced-together discipline made Caycedo's name, but he was unhappy with many of the ways Sophrology was used by practitioners and their different interpretations of it. He went on to found Caycedian Sophrology in order to, "Protect the authenticity of what I created."

Perhaps it's not for us to criticise the great man, but we do disagree with him here. The original yoga tradition has developed many different forms over time. And indeed inspired parts of Sophrology.

It's a testimony to what Caycedo created, that the professional discipline of Sophrology can be tested and has now been officially accepted in many countries. Your author was trained in France and has the RNCP (Répertoire National des Certifications Professionnelles) qualification. The French government added this to their list of professional diplomas in 2012.

The Sophrology presented here has been accepted by the French state and is directly linked to what Caycedo developed.

If this book sparks your interest in Sophrology, don't hesitate to try out different forms with different Sophrologists, to find the one that fits you best. Just like you might try different forms of meditation and yoga.

SOURCES AND INSPIRATIONS

1. Aliotta, Catherine: Manuel de Sophrologie. Fondements, Concepts et Pratique du Métier. 2018, Intereditions.
2. Antiglio, Dominique: The Life-Changing Power of Sophrology. 2018, Yellow Kite.
3. Birbaumer, Niels: Your brain knows more than you think. The New Frontiers of Neuroplasticity. 2014, Ullstein Verlag.
4. Chéné, Patrick-André: Sophrologie, Fondements & Méthodologie, Tome 1. 2018, Edition Ellébore.
5. Hoobyar, Tom, Dotz, Tom: NLP - The Essential Guide to Neurolinguistic Programming. 1994, Harper Collins.
6. Kahneman, Daniel: Thinking Fast and Slow. 2012, Penguin.
7. Seligman, Martin: Authentic Happiness. Using the New Positive Psychology to Realize Your Potential for Lasting Fulfillment. 2004, Atria Books.
8. Courtney E. Ackerman: «What is self confidence? Plus 9 ways to increase it.» https://positivepsychology.com/self-confidence/ November 2019
9. Jeffrey Bernstein: «The two words behind most fears.» https://www.psychologytoday.com/us/blog/liking-the-child-you-love/201909/the-two-words-behind-most-fears September 2019
10. Ed Diener: «Mindfulness and positive thinking.» https://www.pursuit-of-happiness.org/science-of-happiness/positive-thinking/
11. Melanie Greenberg: «9 ways to calm your anxious mind.» https://www.psychologytoday.com/us/blog/the-mindful-self-express/201506/9-ways-calm-your-anxious-mind June 2015
12. William R. Klemm: «12 ways to improve concentration.» https://www.psychologytoday.com/us/blog/memory-medic/201102/12-ways-improve-concentration Febuary 2011
13. Robert L. Leahy: «What is productive worry?» https://www.psychologytoday.com/us/blog/anxiety-files/200805/what-is-productive-worry May 2008
14. Srini Pillay: «The thinking benefits of doodling.» https://www.health.harvard.edu/blog/the-thinking-benefits-of-doodling-2016121510844 December 2016

Printed in Great Britain
by Amazon